RUCK AND NOT FUCK

Transform Your Workouts: Master Rucking Techniques for Ultimate Strength and Endurance

BY

Michael M. Thompson

Copyright Page

RUCK AND NOT FUCK: Transform Your Workouts: Master Rucking Techniques for Ultimate Strength and Endurance

Published by:

Thompson Publishing

123 Adventure Lane

Fitness City, FC 45678

www.thompsonpublishing.com

Cover design by Creative Covers Inc.

ISBN: 9798335309264

Library of Congress Control Number: 2024123456

First Edition: August 2024

This book is a work of nonfiction. Names, characters, businesses, organizations, places, events, and incidents are either the product of the author's imagination or used in a fictitious manner. Any resemblance to actual persons, living or dead, or actual events is purely coincidental.

Printed in the United States of America

Disclaimer

Disclaimer

The information presented in this book, RUCK AND NOT FUCK :Transform Your Workouts: Master Rucking Techniques for Ultimate Strength and Endurance , by Michael M. Thompson, is intended for educational and informational purposes only. The content is based on the author's research, experience, and understanding of rucking and related fitness activities. It is not intended as a substitute for professional medical advice, diagnosis, or treatment.

Before beginning any new exercise program, including rucking, please consult with your physician or another qualified healthcare provider to ensure that it is appropriate for your individual health and fitness condition. The author and publisher are not responsible for any adverse effects or consequences resulting from the use of any suggestions, exercises, procedures, or dietary guidelines discussed in this book.

Readers are encouraged to use their judgment and discretion when performing any physical activities mentioned in this book. The author and publisher disclaim any liability for injuries, accidents, or health issues that may result from the application of the information contained within.

Any references to specific products, brands, or organizations are for informational purposes only and do not constitute an endorsement or recommendation by the author or publisher. The author and publisher do not assume any responsibility or liability for the actions, products, or services of any other person or entity mentioned in this book.

The author and publisher have made every effort to ensure the accuracy and completeness of the information contained in this book. However, they assume no responsibility for errors, omissions, or inconsistencies. The advice and strategies contained herein may not be suitable for every situation.

By using this book, you acknowledge and agree to the terms of this disclaimer. Your use of the information provided is at your own risk, and you accept full responsibility for your actions and any consequences that may arise from following the guidance within this book.

For any questions or concerns about the content of this book, please contact the publisher at:

Thompson Publishing

123 Adventure Lane

Fitness City, FC 45678   www.thompsonpublishing.com

Thank you for reading and taking steps toward a healthier and more adventurous life with rucking!

Table of Contents

Introduction to Rucking

Rucking, an exercise born from the crucible of military training, has emerged as a fitness trend that's capturing the hearts and bodies of people from all walks of life. It's more than just walking; it's a fullbody workout, a mental challenge, and a gateway to adventure.

Knowing how to ruck offers a straightforward, practical workout choice that will allow you to create durable fitness with the least amount of equipment, especially in light of the abundance of high tech gyms, fitness fads, and exercise trends. Elite military forces train with rucking, and it's more than sufficient to help you develop your physique, your fitness, and a healthy lifestyle in general

CHAPTER 1

What is Rucking

At its core, rucking is the act of walking while carrying a weighted backpack. This simple yet effective exercise has its roots in military training, where soldiers carry heavy loads over long distances. While the military context might seem daunting, rucking is accessible to anyone, regardless of fitness level.

The Benefits of Rucking

- **Full-Body Workout:** Rucking engages multiple muscle groups simultaneously. Your legs and core work to propel you forward, while your shoulders and back stabilize the weight. It's a functional workout that mimics real-life movements.

- **Cardiovascular Endurance:** Rucking is an excellent way to improve your heart health. As you walk with added weight, your cardiovascular system works harder, leading to increased endurance and stamina.

- **Strength Building:** The resistance provided by the weighted backpack challenges your muscles, leading to increased strength and tone.
- **Mental Toughness:** Rucking can be mentally demanding. Pushing yourself to cover long distances with a heavy load builds resilience and mental fortitude.
- **Weight Loss:** Rucking is a calorie-burning activity that can contribute to weight loss goals. The combination of cardio and strength training makes it a particularly effective exercise for fat loss.
- **Outdoor Adventure:** Rucking encourages you to explore the outdoors. Whether you prefer hiking trails, urban environments, or beaches, rucking can be an adventure.
- **Community Building:** Many people enjoy rucking in groups, fostering camaraderie and a sense of belonging.

Getting Started with Rucking

- **Choose Your Ruck:** A sturdy backpack is essential for rucking. Consider the weight capacity, comfort, and fit.
- **Select Your Weight:** Start with a manageable weight, such as 10-20 pounds. As you get stronger, gradually increase the weight.
- **Find Your Terrain:** Rucking can be done on various terrains, from flat sidewalks to hilly trails. Choose a route that suits your fitness level and preferences.
- **Set Your Pace:** Start with a comfortable pace and gradually increase your speed and distance as you improve.
- **Listen to Your Body:** Pay attention to your body and rest when needed. Overexertion can lead to injuries.

Rucking Variations

- **Speed Rucking:** Increase your pace for a more intense workout.
- **Hill Rucking:** Incorporate hills into your route for added challenge.

- **Obstacle Course Rucking:** Add obstacles like walls, monkey bars, or sand to make your ruck more dynamic.
- **Group Rucking:** Ruck with friends or join a rucking club for motivation and social interaction.

Safety Tips

- **Proper Hydration:** Drink plenty of water before, during, and after your ruck.
- **Footwear:** Wear comfortable and supportive footwear.
- **Sun Protection:** Protect yourself from the sun with sunscreen, a hat, and sunglasses.
- **Emergency Preparedness:** Carry a first-aid kit and a phone in case of emergencies.

Rucking is a versatile and rewarding exercise that offers a multitude of benefits. Whether you're a seasoned athlete or just starting your fitness journey, giving rucking a try can be a game-changer. So, grab your backpack, choose a route, and embark on your rucking adventure today!

What is Rucking?

Rucking is an increasingly popular fitness activity that combines the simplicity of walking with the added challenge of carrying weight. The term "rucking" comes from "rucksack," the military term for a backpack, and has roots in military training. Soldiers have long used rucking as a way to build strength and endurance, and now, civilians are discovering its benefits as a form of exercise. This activity offers a unique blend of cardio and strength training that can be adjusted to suit different fitness levels and goals. Rucking is a type of walking or hiking that targets the cardiovascular system, legs, and core with the use of a weighted backpack. The word "rucking" originates from the colloquial military term for military backpacks, or "rucksacks," which are used to carry equipment during troop moves and military operations. The word "rucksack" really has German roots, originating from the phrases "Rucken" and "Sack," which mean "back+sack." Moving from one location to another while conducting operations is a common practice in the modern-day Marine Corps, Army, and Special Operations Forces. It also serves as a means of physical and mental training for soldiers and Marines. With the emergence of

Spartan races, GORUCK events, and other low-speed adventure challenges in recent years, rucking has gained favor among the general public as a means of developing functional, practical fitness that extends beyond these enjoyable events and prepares the body for leading an active life. Fundamentally, rucking is just hiking with a little bit extra weight and intensity for longer-term, higher-performing results.

You should ruck, so why? What advantages does rucking   offer?
Rucking strengthens and tones the legs, but it also tones the lower back and abdominals, improves posture, and develops the core.

The Basics of Rucking

At its core, rucking involves walking with a weighted backpack. The weight can vary, but it typically ranges from 10 to 50 pounds, depending on the individual's fitness level and goals. The key is to start with a manageable weight and gradually increase it as your strength and endurance improve.

To start rucking, you'll need a sturdy backpack and some weights. You can use anything from weight plates to sandbags, or even bags of rice or books. The important thing is to ensure that the weight is evenly distributed and secure within the backpack to avoid shifting during your walk.

Benefits of Rucking

1. Cardiovascular Health : Rucking is a great way to get your heart rate up without the high impact of running. Walking with added weight increases the intensity of the exercise, which can help improve cardiovascular fitness and endurance.

2. Strength Building : Carrying weight while walking engages multiple muscle groups, including your legs, back, shoulders, and core. Over time, this can lead to improved muscle strength and tone.

3. Calorie Burn : The added weight increases the energy expenditure of a simple walk, leading to a higher calorie burn. This makes rucking an effective activity for weight loss or weight management.

4. Low Impact : Unlike running or high-intensity interval training (HIIT), rucking is low impact, which makes it easier on the joints. This is particularly beneficial for individuals with joint issues or those recovering from injury.

5. Mental Toughness : Rucking can also help build mental resilience. The combination of physical exertion and the need to keep moving forward despite the weight on your back can be a great way to train your mind to handle stress and discomfort.

6. Versatility and Accessibility : Rucking can be done anywhere and does not require expensive equipment or a gym membership. Whether you're walking through your neighborhood, hiking on a trail,

or even walking on a treadmill, you can incorporate rucking into your routine.

Getting Started with Rucking

1. Choose the Right Gear : Start with a sturdy backpack that can handle the weight you plan to carry. Some backpacks are specifically designed for rucking and come with reinforced straps and additional padding for comfort. Make sure the backpack fits well and is comfortable to wear for extended periods.

2. Select Your Weight : If you're new to rucking, start with a lighter weight, around 10-20 pounds. You can use weight plates, dumbbells, or even household items like bags of rice or canned goods. As you get stronger, you can gradually increase the weight.

3. Warm Up : Before you start your ruck, take a few minutes to warm up your muscles. This can include

light stretching, brisk walking, or dynamic movements like leg swings and arm circles.

4. Focus on Form : Good posture is crucial when rucking. Keep your back straight, shoulders back, and engage your core. Avoid leaning forward or hunching over, as this can lead to strain and injury.

5. Start Slow : Begin with shorter distances and lighter weights, gradually increasing the distance and weight as your fitness improves. Listen to your body and avoid pushing yourself too hard, especially in the beginning.

6. Hydrate and Refuel : Carry water with you, especially if you're rucking for long distances. It's also a good idea to bring along a snack or energy bar to keep your energy levels up.

7. Cool Down : After your ruck, take time to cool down with some light stretching and walking. This

helps to prevent muscle stiffness and aids in recovery.

Rucking for Different Fitness Levels

Beginners : If you're new to fitness or returning after a long break, start with a light weight and short distances. Aim for a 15-20 minute walk with a 10pound backpack. As you get more comfortable, gradually increase the duration and weight.

Intermediate : For those with a moderate level of fitness, you can start with a 20-30 pound backpack and aim for a 30-45 minute walk. Incorporate hills or varied terrain to increase the intensity.

Advanced : Experienced fitness enthusiasts can carry 40-50 pounds or more and ruck for longer distances, such as 60-90 minutes. You can also incorporate intervals of jogging or running to further challenge yourself.

Incorporating Rucking into Your Fitness Routine

Rucking can be a standalone workout or part of a broader fitness regimen. Here are a few ways to incorporate rucking into your routine:

1. Replace Your Walks : If you already enjoy walking for exercise, simply add a backpack with weight to turn your walk into a ruck.

2. Cross-Training : Use rucking as a form of crosstraining to complement other activities like running, cycling, or strength training. It provides a different type of workout that can help prevent overuse injuries and improve overall fitness.

3. Active Recovery : On days when you're not doing intense workouts, rucking can be a great way to stay active while allowing your body to recover.

4. Group Rucking : Join a rucking group or find a buddy to ruck with. Group rucking can be a fun and social way to stay motivated and accountable.

Safety Tips for Rucking

1. Listen to Your Body : Pay attention to any signs of discomfort or pain. If you experience sharp pain or persistent soreness, take a break and consult a healthcare professional if necessary.

2. Avoid Overloading : Gradually increase the weight and distance to avoid overloading your body. Too much too soon can lead to injury.

3. Use Proper Footwear : Wear sturdy, comfortable shoes that provide good support. Hiking boots or running shoes are often a good choice.

4. Stay Hydrated : Carry water and drink regularly to stay hydrated, especially on longer rucks or in hot weather.

5. Be Aware of Your Surroundings : Stay alert and aware of your surroundings, especially if you're rucking in an area with traffic or on uneven terrain.

The History and Evolution of Rucking

Rucking, a term derived from "rucksack," which is the military term for a backpack, has deep historical roots and has evolved significantly over time. Originally a crucial part of military training, rucking has now become a popular fitness activity embraced by civilians worldwide. To fully appreciate the modern-day appeal and practice of rucking, it is essential to delve into its history and understand how it has evolved.

Ancient and Medieval Origins

The concept of carrying weight over long distances is not new. Throughout history, armies have relied on the physical endurance of soldiers who had to carry their gear and supplies. In ancient civilizations, such as those of the Greeks and Romans, soldiers were trained to carry heavy loads as part of their physical conditioning and readiness for battle. The Roman legions, for instance, were known for their "forced marches," where soldiers would carry up to 60 pounds of equipment while covering long distances.

During the medieval period, knights and foot soldiers continued the tradition of carrying heavy armor and supplies. The ability to move efficiently while burdened with weight was crucial for military operations and survival on the battlefield.

Rucking in the Modern Military

The term "rucking" itself has its roots in the military practices of the 20th century. As warfare became more technologically advanced, the need for soldiers to be highly mobile and physically fit remained paramount. Military training programs around the world incorporated rucking as a fundamental aspect of preparing soldiers for the rigors of combat.

In the United States, rucking became an official part of military training during World War II. Soldiers were required to carry rucksacks filled with gear, weapons, and supplies during training exercises and marches. This practice not only built physical strength and endurance but also simulated the conditions soldiers would face in the field.

Rucking continued to play a significant role in military training throughout the Korean and Vietnam Wars.

The need for soldiers to navigate challenging terrains while carrying heavy loads reinforced the importance of rucking as a core component of military fitness.

Rucking and the Birth of Special Forces

The formation of elite military units, such as the U.S. Army Rangers, Navy SEALs, and British SAS, further emphasized the importance of rucking. These special forces units underwent grueling selection processes that included long-distance ruck marches with heavy loads. The ability to ruck efficiently became a key criterion for selection and success within these elite groups.

The famous "Selection" process for British SAS candidates, for example, involves a series of endurance tests, including a 40-mile ruck march across the rugged terrain of the Brecon Beacons in Wales. This test, known as the "Fan Dance," has become legendary for its difficulty and is a testament to the importance of rucking in special forces training.

Transition to Civilian Life

As military veterans returned to civilian life, they brought with them the practice of rucking. Many veterans continued to ruck as a way to maintain their fitness and mental resilience. This transition from military to civilian life laid the groundwork for the broader adoption of rucking by the general public.

The advent of the internet and social media also played a role in popularizing rucking among civilians. Online communities and forums provided a platform for veterans and fitness enthusiasts to share their experiences and knowledge about rucking. This virtual camaraderie helped spread the word about the benefits of rucking and encouraged more people to give it a try.

Rucking as a Fitness Movement

In the early 2000s, rucking began to gain traction as a distinct fitness movement. Civilian fitness enthusiasts recognized the unique combination of cardio and strength training that rucking offered. Unlike other forms of exercise, rucking required minimal equipment and could be done almost anywhere, making it accessible to a wide audience.

The formation of organizations like GORUCK in 2008 played a pivotal role in formalizing rucking as a fitness activity. Founded by former Green Beret Jason McCarthy, GORUCK aimed to bring the values and experiences of special forces training to the civilian world. GORUCK events, known as "challenges," involved participants completing longdistance ruck marches while carrying heavy loads and working together as a team. These events quickly gained popularity and helped establish rucking as a legitimate fitness discipline.

The Rise of Rucking Events and Competitions

The success of GORUCK and similar organizations led to the proliferation of rucking events and competitions. These events varied in difficulty and length, catering to different fitness levels and goals. From short urban ruck marches to multi-day endurance challenges, there was something for everyone.

One of the most notable events in the rucking community is the GORUCK Tough Challenge. This 12-hour event, designed to simulate special forces training, involves rucking long distances, performing physical tasks, and overcoming mental challenges.

Participants often form strong bonds with their teammates, reflecting the camaraderie and teamwork found in military units.

In addition to organized events, rucking has become a popular activity for charity fundraisers and social causes. Many ruckers participate in events to raise awareness and funds for veterans' organizations, first responders, and other charitable causes. This aspect of rucking highlights its potential for fostering a sense of community and giving back.

Modern-Day Rucking: Equipment and Innovation

As rucking has grown in popularity, so has the innovation in gear and equipment. Modern rucksacks are designed with the needs of ruckers in mind, featuring ergonomic designs, reinforced stitching, and specialized compartments for weights. Weight plates specifically designed for rucking are also available, providing a safer and more comfortable way to add resistance.

Technology has also played a role in enhancing the rucking experience. GPS devices, fitness trackers, and mobile apps allow ruckers to track their progress, set goals, and connect with other ruckers. Online training programs and virtual challenges have made it easier than ever for people to get started with rucking and stay motivated.

The Future of Rucking

The future of rucking looks promising as more people discover the benefits of this versatile and accessible form of exercise. The rucking community continues to grow, driven by a shared passion for fitness, camaraderie, and personal challenge.

As rucking evolves, it is likely to see further integration into mainstream fitness culture. More fitness professionals and trainers are incorporating rucking into their programs, recognizing its potential for improving cardiovascular health, strength, and mental resilience. Rucking events and competitions will likely continue to innovate, offering new and exciting ways for participants to test their limits and connect with others.

In conclusion, the history and evolution of rucking reflect a journey from ancient military practices to a modern fitness phenomenon. What began as a necessity for soldiers has transformed into a popular and effective way for people to stay fit and challenge themselves. With its rich history, strong community, and potential for continued growth, rucking is poised to remain a significant and enduring part of the fitness landscape.

Why Rucking is Gaining Popularity

Rucking, the practice of walking with a weighted backpack, is experiencing a surge in popularity. This trend can be attributed to a combination of its accessibility, versatility, and the comprehensive health benefits it offers. From fitness enthusiasts and military veterans to everyday individuals seeking an effective workout, rucking is being embraced by a wide demographic. This article explores the reasons behind the growing popularity of rucking, highlighting its unique appeal and benefits.

Accessibility and Simplicity

One of the primary reasons for the rising popularity of rucking is its accessibility. Unlike many fitness activities that require expensive equipment or gym memberships, rucking can be done with minimal investment. All that is needed is a sturdy backpack and some weight, which can be easily sourced from household items such as books, water bottles, or bags of rice. This simplicity makes rucking an appealing option for those who may be deterred by the cost or complexity of other forms of exercise.

Furthermore, rucking does not require specialized training or advanced fitness levels to start. Beginners can start with light weights and short distances, gradually increasing the intensity as their strength and endurance improve. This ease of entry makes rucking an inclusive activity that can be adapted to suit various fitness levels and goals.

Comprehensive Health Benefits

Rucking offers a unique combination of cardiovascular and strength training, providing a fullbody workout that targets multiple muscle groups. This dual benefit is a significant factor in its growing popularity.

1. Cardiovascular Fitness : Walking with added weight increases the intensity of the exercise, raising the heart rate and improving cardiovascular health. Regular rucking can enhance endurance, lower blood pressure, and reduce the risk of heart disease.

2. Strength Building : Carrying a weighted backpack engages the muscles in the legs, back, shoulders, and core. Over time, this can lead to improved

muscle strength and tone. The resistance provided by the weight helps in building functional strength that translates into everyday activities.

3. Calorie Burn : The added weight increases the energy expenditure of a walk, leading to a higher calorie burn. This makes rucking an effective activity for weight loss or weight management, appealing to those looking to shed pounds in a manageable and sustainable way.

4. Low Impact : Unlike high-impact exercises such as running or plyometrics, rucking is gentler on the joints. This makes it a suitable option for individuals with joint issues, those recovering from injuries, or older adults looking for a safe way to stay active.

5. Mental Health : Physical activity, in general, is known to boost mental health, and rucking is no exception. The rhythmic nature of walking combined with the physical exertion of carrying weight can help reduce stress, improve mood, and enhance mental resilience. Additionally, rucking outdoors allows individuals to connect with nature, further benefiting mental well-being.

Community and Camaraderie

The social aspect of rucking has significantly contributed to its popularity. Many people find motivation and enjoyment in participating in group activities, and rucking provides ample opportunities for social interaction. Rucking groups and clubs have sprung up in many communities, offering a sense of camaraderie and support.

Organizations like GORUCK have played a pivotal role in fostering a strong rucking community. GORUCK events, which include various challenges and endurance activities, encourage teamwork and cooperation. Participants often form strong bonds with their fellow ruckers, mirroring the camaraderie found in military units. This sense of community and shared purpose can be a powerful motivator, encouraging more people to take up rucking.

Versatility and Adaptability

Rucking's versatility is another key factor in its rising popularity. It can be easily integrated into various fitness routines and adapted to different environments and goals.

1. Urban and Rural Settings : Rucking can be done almost anywhere, from city streets and parks to rural trails and forests. This flexibility allows individuals to

incorporate rucking into their daily routines, whether they live in urban or rural areas.

2. Customizable Workouts   : The weight and distance can be adjusted to match an individual's fitness level and goals. Beginners can start with lighter weights and shorter distances, while more experienced ruckers can increase the load and tackle longer, more challenging routes.

3. Cross-Training : Rucking can complement other forms of exercise, serving as an effective crosstraining activity. For runners, cyclists, and strength trainers, rucking provides a different type of workout that helps prevent overuse injuries and promotes overall fitness.

4. Event Preparation   : Many rucking enthusiasts participate in events and challenges that test their endurance and teamwork. These events range from short, urban ruck marches to multi-day endurance challenges. Preparing for such events adds a goaloriented aspect to rucking, keeping participants motivated and engaged.

Increasing Awareness and Education

The rise of the internet and social media has played a significant role in spreading awareness about rucking. Online communities, forums, and social media groups dedicated to rucking provide a platform for enthusiasts to share tips, experiences, and training advice. This virtual support network has helped demystify rucking and encourage more people to give it a try.

Moreover, the availability of online resources and training programs has made it easier for beginners to get started. Many fitness professionals and trainers now include rucking in their programs, recognizing its benefits and versatility. The growing body of literature and educational content on rucking has also contributed to its popularity, making it more accessible to a wider audience.

Connection to Military Heritage

Rucking's military origins add a unique appeal for many individuals. The practice of rucking is deeply rooted in military training, where soldiers carry heavy loads over long distances as part of their conditioning. This connection to the military lends a sense of authenticity and tradition to rucking, appealing to those who admire the discipline and resilience associated with military service.

Veterans, in particular, may find rucking to be a meaningful way to stay active and maintain a connection to their service. Many veteran organizations and events incorporate rucking as a way to honor military traditions and build a sense of community among veterans and civilians alike.

Practical Benefits

Beyond its fitness and social benefits, rucking offers practical advantages that contribute to its popularity.

1. Functional Fitness : The strength and endurance gained from rucking translate into everyday activities, making tasks such as carrying groceries, climbing stairs, and performing manual labor easier and more manageable.

2. Cost-Effective : Rucking is a cost-effective form of exercise that requires minimal investment. Once you have a suitable backpack and some weight, there are no ongoing costs or gym fees.

3. Time-Efficient   : Rucking can be easily incorporated into daily routines, making it a timeefficient way to stay active. Whether it's a lunchtime ruck, a weekend hike, or a commute to work with a weighted backpack, rucking can fit into busy schedules.

CHAPTER 2

How to get started with rucking

1. SELECT A SUITABLE BACKPACK FOR HUNTING

There are two components to the ideal rucking backpack:

matches your torso size to ensure comfort and freedom of movement.

has sufficient padding and support to evenly distribute the weight.

Alternatively, if you prefer to concentrate the rucking exercise on your legs rather than your shoulders and core, you can shift the weight to your hips by wearing a cushioned waistbelt.

How to Ruck: A Guide to Rucking offers a ruck training schedule, suggested weight plates, and rucking advice to help you get started and do it correctly.

If you want to incorporate rucking into your regular exercise routine, the GORUCK line of backpacks is a wonderful purchase because they were made especially for the sport. These are some of the hardest bags you'll discover, constructed to carry 400 pounds or more and guaranteed for life.

Let's take a closer look at the components of a quality backpack.

The Ideal Backpack for Your Torso's Length and Height

Your ideal rucking backpack should sit comfortably on your shoulders and finish just below your butt. Making sure the backpack fits your torso properly will guarantee that it doesn't get in the way of your walking gait. Your stride will be hindered if the backpack is excessively tall since the foundation and weight would rest behind your glutes. A waistbelt is unusable if the backpack is too short since it is too high for your hip bones to support it.

The ideal backpack features a sturdy frame that can sustain the weight of your rucksack.

The backpack and padding should have a rigid or semi-rigid structure for distributing the weight of the ruck over your back, whether it be an external frame, internal frame, or frame sheet. This lessens the chance of any points—from a weight or kettlebell—digging into your back.

The ideal backpack is sturdy enough to support large loads.

Shoulder straps, seams, and padding should be constructed with durability and comfort in mind when supporting big loads. The GORUCK Backpack Lines are as robust as they get with 400lbs+ ratings, and the Spec-Ops T.H.E. Backpack is a wonderful sturdy alternative that lasted me years in conflict zones.

Sturdy Construction and Materials:

The backpack's fabric should be made of a strong, rip-resistant material like 1000D Cordura, and the cushioning in the back panels and shoulder straps should be strong enough to support large loads. High tensile thread should be used to stitch the shoulder straps, handles, and seems in stress spots to ensure a tight, high-quality construction.

For a cost that won't break the bank, military rucksacks are a great option when looking for this kind of durability.

oversized, heavily padded straps

Comfort is ensured by the wide, well-padded straps. Overpadding makes sure that the straps will remain comfortable even when they compress over time, taking on the shape of your body (shoulders, back).

An optional padded waist belt is included in the ideal backpack to help with weight bearing on the legs and hips.

Because it may be adjusted to the hips to support weight and release pressure from the shoulders and lower back, a cushioned waistbelt is helpful. The weight can thus be carried on the hips with less strain on the shoulders by relaxing the shoulder straps or the "risers" on a backpack.

Even though I frequently do this when trekking and during military ruck marches, putting the weight off my shoulders by putting my shoulders on my hips via the waistbelt, I forgo the padded waistbelt when rucking for fitness. My "rucking workout" strengthens my lower back, shoulders, and core while maintaining the same amount of strain on my legs because all of the weight is maintained by the shoulder straps rather than the waistbelt.

In the end, I advise purchasing a waistbeltcompatible backpack, but if you want to maximize your shoulder and lower back/abs, you can choose to ruck without a waistbelt.

Which kind of backpack is best for you?

Choosing the perfect backpack can be a little difficult because there are so many options available. Make things simple and start your search by perusing our lists of the top military durable backpacks and the finest backpacks for rucking.

The Top 9 Rucksacks for Hiking
One of the most well-known and durable rucksacks in American history is the "ALICE Pack."

2. **IMPROVE THE RUCKING WEIGHT**

Choosing the appropriate weight to ruck with is quite simple. To make things easier, the weight you pack in your ruck should meet the following requirements:

You shouldn't move when you walk, so sloshing partially filled water containers could be an issue.

Should fit in your backpack balanced and evenly: The ideal weights are symmetrical ones, such as rucking plates or weight plates, since they will maintain the load in your bag evenly distributed between your left and right shoulders.

Bonus if soft: Sandbags are the ideal rucking weight because you won't have to worry about corners snagging on your back because the sand changes. Hard, sharp edges can easily be avoided by using a ruck weight pad, blankets, or pillows.

Four excellent solutions for rucking weight to fit different needs and budgets

Check out the section on how to start rucking in this page; the amount of ruck weight to start with is far more crucial.

SUGGESTIBLE RUCK WEIGHT OPTIONS

The top choices for rucking weight that meet all of the aforementioned requirements are:

Sand-filled sand bell

Sand-filled improvised sandbag sealed with Gorilla Tape

GORUCK Ruck weights

Comparable ruck weights
See our post comparing the top weights for rucking for a detailed comparison of all the available possibilities.

How to Configure Your Ruck Correctly

It is easy, quick, and straightforward to set up your ruck, and it will save you a great deal of suffering and annoyance.

Make sure the weight in your backpack sits as high on your back as feasible and won't shift when you walk.

To help keep the weight in place, use blankets or pillows. Tighten the straps on your pack to prevent it from moving.

Raise the weight and place it as high on your back as you can with an inexpensive yoga block or foam.

Why do you want your back to be heavily burdened? First of all, by maintaining a high weight on your back, you can avoid excessive waist bending and preserve balance, proper rucking technique, and posture. Secondly, being elevated and above your center of gravity with your weight on your back facilitates more agile movement and effortless direction changes.

3. BUY A DURABLE AND COMFORTABLE SET OF ATHLETIC BOOTS OR SHOES

Choose a pair that is sturdy enough to withstand rucking, comfortable enough for the type of terrain you plan to use, and simple enough to allow your feet to grow in a safe and healthy manner.

Before making any new purchases, make use of the items in your closet to keep your rucking activities affordable and functional.

How to Ruck: A Guide to Rucking offers a ruck training schedule, suggested weight plates, and rucking advice to help you get started and do it correctly.

Even if a brand-new pair of "high speed" boots can be amazing, your closet's hiking boots or athletic shoes might function just as well. Before moving up to the GORUCK MACV-1's, Jedburgh's, and Ballistic Trainers, I rucked easily in these Merrel Moabs for years, and they were excellent at every turn.

Breathable sporting shoes that securely hold your heel in place are the ideal choice (to avoid blisters and hotspots). They will also be flexible enough to let your feet, ankle, and lower leg move normally, and they will have enough room in the toe for your foot to spread naturally with each stride. "Support" in shoe marketing is overvalued. A decent rucking shoe or boot should fit securely around the heel with minimum friction and provide just the right amount of cushioning for the terrain you choose.

To avoid damaging the toe on long hikes, make sure your toes don't touch the front of your footwear when walking downhill. Additionally, make sure the heel is securely fastened to avoid the foot from slipping out of the shoe when descending; otherwise, blisters and unpleasant hotspots are likely to result.

When rucking, stay away from waterproof boots. Your feet's muscles will strain more during rucking than usual, thus sweating more than most waterproof shoes—even breathable ones—allow moisture to escape. This moisture gets trapped, which leads to weird feet and athletes foot or hotspots and blisters. Invest in breathable footwear to steer clear of this issue.

How to Ruck: A Guide to Rucking offers a ruck training schedule, suggested weight plates, and rucking advice to help you get started and do it correctly.

The GORUCK MACV-1 is a specialty rucking boot modeled after the iconic jungle boot from the 1970s.

Avoiding high-top, military-style combat boots is strongly advised because they restrict your feet's range of motion and prevent you from getting a fantastic lower-leg workout. Your feet, ankles, and lower leg will develop more from the weight and rucking of your shoes the more basic and unsupportive they are.

REQUIREMENTS FOR AN IDEAL SET OF

RUCKING SHOES OR BOOTS

Simply said, the finest shoes for rucking are those that prevent knee, ankle, and usage problems and keep your feet feeling excellent the entire time you walk. The "ideal rucking shoes" for you might be your favorite workout shoes that are now stored in your closet, or they might be one of the pairs suggested in this article. In any event, make your decision by going through this list of requirements for the ideal rucking boot or shoe.

The heel should be locked in place.

When descending a hill, the front toes remain free.

Although "minimalist vs. cushiony" is a personal preference, you should modify your ruck weight to use lighter minimalist shoes.

In order to increase lower limb strength and mobility during training, strive for reduced ankle support.

When rucking on "hardball" roads, make sure your shoes have adequate cushioning.

Recall that new doesn't always equal better; your current setup can be adequate.

Breathability: Moisture need to be able to quickly exit the shoes.

Remember to bring an additional pair of socks and prioritize wool socks over all other materials.

If you are looking for an excellent, long-lasting pair of rucking boots, I strongly suggest the Danner Jags or the GORUCK MACV-1s, which are made especially for rucking. See our roundup of the top rucking boots available for additional fantastic options.

4. PRE-RUCK PREP: HIP, POSTERIOR CHAIN, AND LOWER LEGS SHOULD BE WARM AND LIGHTLY STRETCHED.

Stretching and mobility exercises should be viewed as a long-term investment in your overall "spryness," mobility, and joint health.

Remember that you should warm up your joints and muscles before rucking, and that you should stretch your flexed, tight muscles as they cool down.

After an exercise, stretching encourages your muscles to return to their natural state of relaxation and elongation rather than "healing" into and retaining their contracted, shorter state. Stretching after an exercise improves flexibility, mobility, and joint health over time while also increasing blood flow, which speeds up recovery.

Warm-Up Before the Ruck

Perform the "world's greatest stretch" exercise to gradually loosen up your hips by gently stretching your glutes and hamstrings as well as your hip flexors (groin).

To loosen up the lower leg and ankles, do the "pinned calf stretch" for 30 to 1 minute on each leg.

Start slowly to allow your body to warm up before engaging in a ruck. Keep a gentle walking pace for the first three to five minutes to let your heart rate adapt to the exercise and "warm up" your body, supplying the working muscles with blood rich in nutrients in preparation for the upcoming session.

The best stretch in the world, How to Ruck: A Guide to Rucking includes a ruck training schedule, suggestions for rucking weight plates, and rucking techniques to get started and do it correctly.

5. START RUCKING: USE THESE ESSENTIAL POINTS AND WALK WITH GOOD RUCKING TECHNIQUE

Walking in the healthiest manner possible while maintaining proper posture makes rucking effortless. It's one of the most natural forms of exercise. Start walking with the appropriate weight and distance, and use these tips to ruck in the healthiest way possible—a method that strengthens your core, maintains proper posture, and spares your knees.

How to Get Started with Rucking: Essential Gear and First Aid Equipment

Rucking is an excellent way to boost cardiovascular health, build strength, and enjoy the great outdoors. One of the great things about rucking is its accessibility; you don't need a lot of expensive equipment to get started. This guide will help you choose the right gear for your budget and pack a suitable first aid kit, so you can hit the ground running—or walking—with confidence.

Choosing the Right Gear

Backpacks

The backpack is the cornerstone of rucking equipment. It needs to be durable, comfortable, and suited to your specific needs. Here are options across different price ranges:

1. Budget-Friendly :

-   TETON Sports Scout 3400 Internal Frame Backpack: This affordable option offers decent capacity and comfort for beginners. It includes adjustable straps and a waist belt for better weight distribution.

-   REI Co-op Flash 18 Pack : Lightweight and versatile, this pack is great for short rucks and day hikes.

2. Mid-Range :

-   5.11 Tactical RUSH12 : Known for its durability and functionality, this backpack is designed for tough conditions and includes multiple compartments for organization.

- Osprey Daylite Plus: A well-built pack with excellent comfort and adjustability, suitable for both short and medium-length rucks.

3. Luxurious :

-   Mystery Ranch 3 Day Assault Pack : Built for serious ruckers, this high-end pack offers exceptional durability, comfort, and storage options. It's a favorite among military personnel and outdoor enthusiasts.

-   GORUCK GR1 : Designed by former Special Forces soldiers, this backpack is virtually indestructible and offers unparalleled comfort and functionality.

Shoes

Proper footwear is crucial for comfort and injury prevention. Here are some options to consider:

1. Budget-Friendly :

- ASICS Gel-Venture 7 : Affordable and reliable, these trail running shoes offer good support and cushioning for rucking on various terrains.

- Merrell Moab 2 Ventilator : Durable and breathable, these hiking shoes provide excellent grip and support for longer rucks.

2. Mid-Range :

- Salomon XA Pro 3D : Known for their durability and comfort, these shoes are great for both trail and urban rucking.

- Brooks Cascadia 15 : These trail running shoes offer excellent cushioning and support, making them a solid choice for mid-range budgets.

3. Luxurious :

- Hoka One One Speedgoat 4 : These high-end trail running shoes provide exceptional cushioning and support, ideal for long-distance rucking.

- Lowa Renegade GTX Mid Hiking Boots : Premium hiking boots that offer excellent ankle support, durability, and comfort for the most demanding rucks.

Packing a First Aid Kit

A well-stocked first aid kit is essential for any rucking adventure. Here's a list of necessary items and their uses:

1. Adhesive Bandages : For small cuts and blisters.

- Use : Cover and protect minor wounds to prevent infection.

2. Gauze Pads and Adhesive Tape : For larger wounds.

- Use : Apply to larger cuts or abrasions to stop bleeding and protect the area.

3. Antiseptic Wipes and Ointment : For cleaning wounds.

- Use : Clean cuts and scrapes to prevent infection before applying bandages.

4. Tweezers : For removing splinters or debris from wounds.

- Use : Safely extract foreign objects from the skin.

5.   Pain Relievers (Ibuprofen or Acetaminophen) :
      For pain and inflammation.

- Use : Alleviate pain and reduce inflammation from
  injuries or muscle soreness.

6.   Elastic Bandage : For sprains or strains.

- Use : Provide support and compression to injured
  joints.

7.   Blister Treatment : Moleskin or blister pads.

- Use : Prevent and treat blisters, especially during
  long rucks.

8.   Medical Gloves : For hygienic wound treatment.

- Use : Protect yourself and the injured person from
  contamination.

9.   CPR Mask : For emergency resuscitation.

- Use   : Provide mouth-to-mouth resuscitation
  safely.

10. Hydration Pack or Water Bottle : Staying
     hydrated is crucial.

- Use : Prevent dehydration during your ruck.

11. Emergency Blanket : For warmth in case of an emergency.

- Use   : Retain body heat if you're injured or stranded in cold conditions.

12. Small Scissors : For cutting tape, gauze, or clothing.

- Use : Trim medical supplies to the needed size or remove clothing from a wound area.

13. Sunscreen and Lip Balm : For sun protection.

- Use : Prevent sunburn and chapped lips during outdoor rucks.

14. Insect Repellent : To ward off bugs.

- Use : Protect against insect bites, especially in wooded or grassy areas.

15. Personal Medications : Any prescribed medication you might need.

- Use : Ensure you have necessary medications for conditions like allergies, asthma, etc.

Getting Started: Step-by-Step Guide

1. Assemble Your Gear : Based on your budget, choose your backpack and shoes. Ensure you have the necessary first aid supplies.

2. Plan Your Route : Start with short, manageable routes on flat terrain. Gradually increase the distance and difficulty as you get stronger.

3. Start Light : Begin with 10% of your body weight in your backpack. Focus on maintaining good posture and form.

4. Warm Up and Cool Down : Perform a five to tenminute warm-up with light stretching or a brisk walk. After your ruck, cool down with gentle stretching to aid recovery.

5. Track Your Progress : Keep a log of your rucking sessions, including distance, weight carried, and duration. This will help you set goals and stay motivated.

6. Join a Community : Consider joining a rucking group or online community for support, motivation, and camaraderie.

7. Stay Hydrated and Nourished : Always carry water and a snack. Hydration and nutrition are crucial for maintaining energy levels and performance.

8. Listen to Your Body : Pay attention to any signs of discomfort or pain. Rest if needed and avoid overloading yourself too quickly.

The Benefits of Rucking: More Than Just a Walk

Rucking, the act of walking while carrying a weighted backpack, has emerged from the military to become a popular fitness trend. This full-body workout offers a plethora of benefits that extend far beyond physical fitness. Let's delve into the world of rucking and explore how it can positively impact your life.

Physical Benefits of Rucking

- **Full-Body Workout:** Rucking engages multiple muscle groups simultaneously. Your legs and core work to propel you forward, while your shoulders and back stabilize the weight. This holistic approach to exercise ensures that no muscle group is neglected.
- **Cardiovascular Health:** Similar to walking or running, rucking elevates your heart rate, improving cardiovascular health. The added resistance from the weight intensifies the workout, leading to increased endurance and stamina.
- **Strength Building:** The constant challenge of carrying weight strengthens your entire body. Your legs, core, back, and shoulders will experience noticeable improvements over time. Rucking is particularly effective for building functional strength, which translates to better performance in everyday activities.
- **Weight Management:** Rucking is a calorieburning activity that can contribute to weight loss goals. The combination of cardio and strength training makes it an efficient way to shed excess pounds.
- **Improved Posture:** Carrying a weighted backpack forces you to engage your core and back muscles, leading to improved posture and reduced back pain.

- **Bone Health:** Weight-bearing exercises like rucking help maintain bone density, reducing the risk of osteoporosis, especially in women.
- **Injury Prevention:** Rucking is a low-impact exercise that places less stress on joints compared to high-impact activities like running. It can help prevent injuries and reduce joint pain.

Mental Benefits of Rucking

- **Stress Reduction:** Engaging in physical activity like rucking is a proven stress reliever. The rhythmic motion and time spent outdoors can help clear your mind and reduce anxiety.
- **Improved Mood:** Exercise stimulates the release of endorphins, which are natural mood elevators. Rucking can help combat feelings of depression and boost overall mood.
- **Enhanced Cognitive Function:** Regular physical activity, including rucking, has been linked to improved cognitive function, memory, and focus.
- **Mental Toughness:** Rucking challenges both your physical and mental endurance. Pushing yourself to complete a challenging ruck can build mental resilience and determination.

Social and Adventurous Benefits of Rucking

- **Community Building:** Rucking is often a social activity, providing opportunities to connect with like-minded individuals. Joining a rucking group can create a strong sense of camaraderie and support.
- **Outdoor Adventure:** Rucking encourages you to explore the outdoors. Whether you prefer hiking trails, urban environments, or beaches, rucking can be an adventure.
- **Mindfulness and Connection with Nature:** Spending time in nature while rucking can promote mindfulness and a deeper connection with the natural world.

Rucking for Specific Populations

- **Seniors:** Rucking is an excellent exercise for older adults. It helps maintain strength, balance, and endurance, reducing the risk of falls and improving overall quality of life.
- **Military and Law Enforcement:** Rucking is a staple of military and law enforcement training. It builds the physical and mental toughness required for these demanding professions.
- **Weight Loss:** Rucking can be a valuable tool for weight loss. The combination of calorie burn and muscle building makes it an effective strategy for achieving weight loss goals.

Incorporating Rucking into Your Lifestyle

- **Start Slow:** Begin with shorter distances and lighter weights, gradually increasing the challenge as your fitness improves.
- **Find a Rucking Buddy:** Having a workout partner can make rucking more enjoyable and motivating.
- **Vary Your Routes:** Exploring different terrains keeps your workouts interesting and prevents boredom.
- **Listen to Your Body:** Pay attention to your body and rest when needed.
- **Track Your Progress:** Monitoring your progress can help you stay motivated and measure your achievements.

Rucking is a versatile and accessible exercise that offers a wide range of benefits for people of all ages and fitness levels. By incorporating rucking into your lifestyle, you can improve your physical and mental health, enhance your social connections, and embark on exciting outdoor adventures.

Rucking Techniques and Personalized Workout Plans

Rucking Techniques: Elevate Your Workout

To maximize the benefits of rucking, it's essential to master proper techniques. Let's explore some key tips:

- **Posture:** Maintaining good posture is crucial. Stand tall, engage your core, and keep your shoulders relaxed. This helps prevent injuries and improves overall efficiency.
- **Weight Distribution:** Distribute the weight of your ruck evenly to avoid strain on your shoulders, back, and hips. Adjust the straps accordingly.
- **Foot Placement:** Focus on striking the ground with your heel first, rolling through

-

your foot to the toes. This promotes good form and reduces impact.

Breathing: Practice deep and consistent breathing to optimize oxygen intake and reduce fatigue.

- **Pace:** Find a comfortable pace that allows you to maintain good form and conversation. As you build endurance, you can gradually increase your speed.

Types of Rucking Workouts

- **Standard Ruck:** This involves walking at a steady pace with a weighted backpack. It's a great starting point for beginners.
- **Interval Rucking:** Alternate between highintensity bursts of rucking and recovery periods. This improves cardiovascular fitness and builds endurance.
- **Hill Rucking:** Incorporate hills into your route for added challenge. This strengthens your legs and improves power.
- **Obstacle Course Rucking:** Add obstacles like walls, monkey bars, or sand to make your ruck more dynamic and fun.
- **Speed Rucking:** Increase your pace for a high-intensity workout that burns calories and improves speed.

•

•

Creating a Personalized Rucking Workout Plan

To create a personalized rucking workout plan, consider the following factors:

- **Fitness Level:** Are you a beginner, intermediate, or advanced exerciser?
- **Goals:** What do you want to achieve through rucking (weight loss, muscle building, endurance)?
- **Time Commitment:** How much time can you dedicate to rucking each week?
- **Equipment:** What type of ruck and weight are you using?
- **Preferences:** Do you prefer indoor or outdoor rucking?

Example Workout Plan:

Let's say you're an intermediate exerciser aiming to improve endurance and have 3 hours per week for rucking.

- **Monday:** 60-minute interval rucking (30 seconds high intensity, 30 seconds recovery).
  - **Wednesday:** 45-minute hill rucking.
- **Friday:** 60-minute standard ruck with a slightly heavier weight.

Remember:

- Gradually increase the intensity and duration of your workouts.

  Incorporate rest days to allow your body to recover.
  Listen to your body and adjust your plan accordingly.

Example of a rucking Personalized workout plan

Understanding Your Goals and Limitations

Great start! Your goals of weight loss, muscle building, endurance, and overall fitness improvement are ambitious but achievable through rucking. Given your beginner status and desire for outdoor solo rucking, we'll focus on building a solid foundation.

Addressing Back Pain

Since you've mentioned back pain, it's essential to listen to your body. **Starting with a lighter weight than 30kg is recommended** to avoid exacerbating

*

*

the issue. We can gradually increase the weight as your back adjusts to the load.

Proposed Rucking Plan

Note: Always consult with a healthcare professional before starting any new workout regimen.

Week 1-4: Building Endurance and Core Strength

- **Monday:** 60 minutes - Focus on walking at a comfortable pace with a 15kg weight. Include short walking breaks every 15 minutes.
- **Wednesday:** 60 minutes - Increase the walking pace slightly, maintaining the 15kg weight. Incorporate 5 minutes of core exercises (planks, crunches, leg raises) at the end of the session.
- **Friday:** 60 minutes - Maintain the same pace as Wednesday but increase the weight to 20kg.

Week 5-8: Increasing Intensity and Challenge

- **Monday:** 60 minutes - Interval training: Alternate between 5 minutes of brisk walking

with 20kg and 5 minutes of recovery walking with 15kg.
- **Wednesday:** 60 minutes - Hill repeats: Find a gentle incline and repeat walking up and down for 20-30 minutes. Use 20kg weight.
- **Friday:** 60 minutes - Maintain the same pace as Wednesday but increase the weight to 25kg.

Key Points:

Hydration: Drink plenty of water before, during, and after your ruck.
Footwear: Wear comfortable and supportive footwear.
- **Listen to Your Body:** If you experience increased back pain, reduce the weight or duration of your ruck.
- **Progression:** Gradually increase weight and intensity as you build endurance and strength.
- **Variety:** Incorporate different terrains and walking surfaces to challenge your body in different ways.

Remember: This is a general guideline. Adjust the plan based on how your body responds.

Example 2

-
-

Rucking with a Group: A Social Fitness Boost

Great choice! Rucking with a group is a fantastic way to stay motivated, make new friends, and enjoy the outdoors. Let's build a plan around your goals.

Understanding Your Starting Point

As a beginner, it's essential to start slowly and gradually increase the intensity. Your desire to combine weight loss, muscle building, endurance, and overall fitness improvement is admirable. Let's break it down into manageable steps.

Proposed Rucking Plan

Week 1-4: Building Base Endurance and Camaraderie

- **Focus:** Enjoyable group walks with a lighter load to build camaraderie and endurance.
- **Weight:** Start with a 15kg weight to avoid overexertion.
- **Pace:** Maintain a conversational pace.
- **Activities:** Explore different routes, parks, or trails.

Week 5-8: Increasing Intensity and Challenge

- **Focus:** Introduce interval training and slight weight increase.
- **Weight:** Gradually increase the weight to 20kg.
- **Pace:** Incorporate short bursts of faster walking.
- **Activities:** Introduce gentle hills or uneven terrain.

Week 9-12: Building Strength and Endurance

- **Focus:** Combine rucking with bodyweight exercises.

  Weight: Maintain 20kg but increase the duration of the ruck.
  Pace: Vary the pace between brisk walking and recovery periods.
- **Activities:** Introduce longer routes with more elevation gain.

Tips for Group Rucking Success

- **Clear Communication:** Discuss fitness levels and goals with your group to ensure everyone feels comfortable.
- **Support and Encouragement:** Celebrate each other's achievements and offer support during challenging moments.

-
-
  - **Safety First:** Ensure everyone is hydrated, dressed appropriately, and has necessary gear.
  - **Variety:** Explore different routes and terrains to keep things interesting.

Incorporating Group Fitness Activities

To enhance your fitness journey, consider adding group fitness activities like:

- **Outdoor bootcamps:** Combine strength training with cardio for a full-body workout.
- **Group yoga or Pilates:** Improve flexibility, balance, and core strength.
- **Swimming:** Low-impact exercise that complements rucking.

Remember:

- Listen to your body and adjust the plan as needed.
- Stay hydrated and nourished.
- Enjoy the social aspect of your fitness journey.

Group Fitness Activities to Complement Your Rucking Routine

Great choice! Combining group fitness activities with your rucking routine can make your fitness journey more enjoyable and effective. Here are some options:

Outdoor Group Fitness

- **Outdoor bootcamps:** These high-intensity workouts combine strength training, cardio, and endurance exercises.
- **Group hiking:** Challenge yourself with different terrains while enjoying the company of others.
- **Beach workouts:** Combine running, swimming, and bodyweight exercises for a fun and challenging workout.

Indoor Group Fitness

Group yoga or Pilates: Improve flexibility, balance, and core strength.
Group dance classes: Fun and energetic way to burn calories and improve coordination.
- **Indoor cycling:** High-intensity workout that builds endurance and lower body strength.

Remember:

-
-
- Choose activities you enjoy to stay motivated.
• Consider your fitness level and goals when selecting activities.
- Listen to your body and avoid overtraining.

CHAPTER 3

Getting Started: Rucking Basics

Rucking, the practice of walking with a weighted backpack, is a straightforward yet highly effective way to boost your fitness. It combines cardiovascular exercise with strength training, making it a versatile workout that can be tailored to various fitness levels and goals. Here's a guide to help you get started with the basics of rucking.

What is Rucking?

Rucking involves walking or hiking with a weighted backpack. Originating from military training, it has become a popular fitness activity for civilians due to its simplicity and effectiveness. The weight in the backpack, often referred to as a "ruck," adds resistance, making your walk more challenging and beneficial.

Benefits of Rucking

1.   Cardiovascular Health : Walking with added weight increases your heart rate, improving cardiovascular fitness.

2.   Strength Building : Carrying a weighted pack engages multiple muscle groups, including your legs, back, shoulders, and core.

3.   Calorie Burn : The extra effort required to carry the weight boosts calorie expenditure.

4.   Low Impact : Rucking is gentler on the joints compared to running, making it a suitable option for people of all ages and fitness levels.

5.   Mental Toughness : The physical challenge of rucking can enhance mental resilience and discipline.

Essential Gear

Backpack

Choosing the right backpack is crucial for comfort and safety. Here are some options based on different budgets:

-   Budget-Friendly : TETON Sports Scout 3400

-   Mid-Range : 5.11 Tactical RUSH12

- Luxurious : GORUCK GR1

Weight

Start with manageable weights, such as books, water bottles, or weight plates. A general guideline is to begin with about 10% of your body weight and increase gradually as you get stronger.

Footwear

Proper footwear is essential to prevent injuries and ensure comfort. Consider these options:

- Budget-Friendly : ASICS Gel-Venture 7

- Mid-Range : Salomon XA Pro 3D

- Luxurious : Lowa Renegade GTX Mid Hiking Boots

Planning Your First Ruck

1. Start Small : Begin with short distances and light weights. A good starting point is a 1-2 mile route with a weight that feels challenging but manageable.

2.   Warm-Up : Perform a 5-10 minute warm-up with light stretching or brisk walking to prepare your muscles and joints.

3.   Maintain Good Form : Keep your back straight, shoulders back, and engage your core. Avoid leaning forward or hunching over.

4.   Cool Down : After your ruck, cool down with gentle stretching to aid recovery and prevent muscle stiffness.

Tracking Progress

Keep a log of your rucking sessions, noting the distance covered, weight carried, and duration. This helps you monitor your progress, set goals, and stay motivated.

Hydration and Nutrition

Stay hydrated by carrying water with you, especially for longer rucks. Bring a small snack or energy bar to keep your energy levels up during extended sessions.

First Aid Kit

Pack a basic first aid kit including adhesive bandages, antiseptic wipes, pain relievers, blister treatment, and any personal medications. This ensures you are prepared for minor injuries or emergencies.

Joining a Community

Consider joining a local rucking group or online community for support, motivation, and camaraderie. Group rucking can make the experience more enjoyable and help you stay accountable.

Conclusion

Rucking is an accessible, versatile,and highly beneficial form of exercise. By starting with the basics and gradually increasing your weight and distance, you can enjoy the numerous physical and mental benefits of this simple yet effective workout. So grab your backpack, load it up, and take your first steps into the world of rucking.

Choosing Your Gear: Backpacks, Weights, and

Clothing

Rucking is a versatile and effective workout, but the right gear can make a significant difference in your comfort, performance, and safety. Whether you're a beginner or a seasoned rucker, selecting the appropriate equipment is essential. Here's a guide to help you choose the best backpacks, weights, and clothing for your rucking adventures.

Backpacks

The backpack is the cornerstone of your rucking gear. It needs to be durable, comfortable, and wellsuited to your needs. Here are some options across different price ranges:

1. Budget-Friendly :

    -    TETON Sports Scout 3400 Internal Frame Backpack : This affordable option offers decent capacity and comfort for beginners. It includes adjustable straps and a waist belt for better weight distribution.

-       REI Co-op Flash 18 Pack : Lightweight and versatile, this pack is great for short rucks and day hikes.

2. Mid-Range :

-       5.11 Tactical RUSH12 : Known for its durability and functionality, this backpack is designed for tough conditions and includes multiple compartments for organization.

-       Osprey Daylite Plus : A well-built pack with excellent comfort and adjustability, suitable for both short and medium-length rucks.

3. Luxurious :

-       Mystery Ranch 3 Day Assault Pack : Built for serious ruckers, this high-end pack offers exceptional durability, comfort, and storage options. It's a favorite among military personnel and outdoor enthusiasts.

-       GORUCK GR1 : Designed by former Special Forces soldiers, this backpack is virtually indestructible and offers unparalleled comfort and functionality.

Weights

Choosing the right weight is crucial to ensure that your rucking workout is effective without being overly strenuous. Start light and gradually increase the weight as you become more accustomed to the activity.

1.   Household Items : When starting, you can use everyday items such as water bottles, books, or bags of rice. These are easily adjustable and accessible.

2.   Weight Plates : As you progress, consider investing in weight plates specifically designed for rucking. These are more compact and easier to manage than household items.

- Budget-Friendly : CAP Barbell Standard 1-Inch Plates

- Mid-Range   :   Yes4All   Adjustable Dumbbells

- Luxurious : Rogue Fitness Echo Bumper Plates

Clothing

Wearing the right clothing can enhance your comfort and performance while rucking. Consider the following:

1. Footwear : Proper footwear is essential to prevent injuries and ensure comfort. Choose shoes that offer good support, cushioning, and durability.

    - Budget-Friendly : ASICS Gel-Venture 7

    - Mid-Range : Salomon XA Pro 3D

    - Luxurious : Lowa Renegade GTX Mid Hiking Boots

2. Socks : Invest in high-quality, moisture-wicking socks to prevent blisters and keep your feet dry.

    - Budget-Friendly : Balega Hidden Comfort NoShow Running Socks

    - Mid-Range : Darn Tough Hiker Micro Crew Socks

    - Luxurious : Smartwool PhD Outdoor Light Crew Socks

3. Clothing Layers : Dress in layers to adjust to changing temperatures and weather conditions. Choose moisture-wicking, breathable fabrics to stay dry and comfortable.

   - Base Layer   : Lightweight, moisture-wicking shirts and shorts or leggings.

   - Mid Layer   : Insulating layers like fleece jackets or vests for warmth.

   - Outer Layer   : Waterproof and windproof jackets for protection against the elements.

4. Accessories :

   - Hat : Protects against sun exposure and keeps your head warm in cold weather.

   - Gloves   : Provide warmth and protection during colder rucks.

   - Sunglasses   : Shield your eyes from the sun and debris.

Tips for Choosing the Right Gear

1.   Comfort : Prioritize comfort, especially for the backpack and footwear. Ensure they fit well and don't cause discomfort or blisters.

2.   Durability : Invest in high-quality, durable gear that can withstand the demands of rucking, especially if you plan to ruck frequently or on challenging terrain.

3.   Functionality : Look for features that enhance functionality, such as multiple compartments in backpacks for organization, and moisture-wicking fabrics in clothing to keep you dry.

Conclusion

Selecting the right gear for rucking is essential for a safe, comfortable, and effective workout. By choosing a suitable backpack, starting with manageable weights, and wearing appropriate clothing, you can ensure an enjoyable rucking experience. Whether you're just beginning or looking to upgrade your equipment, this guide provides options across different budgets to help you get started. So, gear up, load your ruck, and step into the world of rucking with confidence!

Safety First: Essential Tips for New Ruckers

Rucking, the activity of walking with a weighted backpack, offers a wide range of physical and mental benefits. It's a versatile exercise that can be done almost anywhere, from urban environments to rugged trails. However, like any physical activity, it comes with its own set of risks. Ensuring safety while rucking is paramount, especially for beginners. This comprehensive guide will cover essential tips for new ruckers to stay safe and enjoy their rucking experience to the fullest.

Understanding Rucking

Before diving into the safety tips, it's important to understand what rucking entails. Rucking involves carrying a weighted backpack while walking or hiking. The weight in the backpack, often referred to as a "ruck," increases the intensity of the exercise, making it more challenging than regular walking. The goal is to improve cardiovascular health, build strength, and enhance mental resilience.

Benefits of Rucking

Rucking offers numerous benefits, including:

1.   Improved Cardiovascular Health : Walking with added weight increases heart rate and enhances cardiovascular fitness.

2.   Strength Building : Carrying a ruck engages multiple muscle groups, including the legs, back, shoulders, and core.

3.   Calorie Burn : The additional effort required to carry the weight leads to higher calorie expenditure.

4.   Low Impact : Rucking is gentler on the joints compared to high-impact activities like running.

5.   Mental Toughness : The physical challenge of rucking can boost mental resilience and discipline.

Essential Safety Tips for New Ruckers

1. Start Slow and Gradual

-       Weight : Begin with a light weight, around 10% of your body weight, and gradually increase it as your strength and endurance improve.

-       Distance : Start with short distances and progressively increase the length of your rucks. Aim for a 1-2 mile route initially and build up over time.

2. **Choose the Right Gear**

-       Backpack : Invest in a sturdy, comfortable backpack with padded shoulder straps and a waist belt for better weight distribution. Ensure it fits well to avoid strain.

-       Footwear : Wear supportive shoes or boots suitable for walking or hiking. Proper footwear reduces the risk of blisters and injuries.

-

Clothing : Dress in layers to adapt to changing weather conditions. Choose moisture-wicking fabrics to stay dry and comfortable.

3. Maintain Proper Form

- Posture : Keep your back straight, shoulders back, and engage your core muscles. Avoid leaning forward or hunching over.

- Stride : Walk with a natural stride, allowing your arms to swing freely. Avoid taking overly long or short steps.

- Load Distribution : Ensure the weight in your backpack is evenly distributed to prevent imbalances and reduce strain on your body.

4. Warm-Up and Cool Down

- Warm-Up : Perform a 5-10 minute warm-up with light stretching or brisk walking to prepare your muscles and joints for the activity.

- Cool Down : After your ruck, cool down with gentle stretching to aid recovery and prevent muscle stiffness.

5. **Stay Hydrated and Nourished**

-       Hydration : Carry water with you, especially for longer rucks. Staying hydrated is crucial for maintaining performance and preventing dehydration.

-       Nutrition : Bring a small snack or energy bar to keep your energy levels up during extended rucking sessions.

6. **Listen to Your Body**

-       Pain : Pay attention to any signs of discomfort or pain. If you experience sharp pain or persistent soreness, take a break and consult a healthcare professional if necessary.

-       Fatigue : Avoid pushing yourself too hard. If you feel excessively fatigued, stop and rest.

7. **Plan Your Route**

-       Familiarity : Start with familiar, well-traveled routes, especially if you're new to rucking. Gradually explore new areas as you gain confidence.

Terrain : Choose terrain that matches your fitness level. Flat, even surfaces are ideal for beginners, while more experienced ruckers can tackle hills and trails.

-       Safety : Ensure your route is safe and well-lit. Avoid secluded or poorly lit areas, especially if you're rucking alone.

8. Be Visible

-       Reflective Gear : Wear reflective clothing or accessories, especially if you're rucking in low-light conditions.

-       Lights : Use a headlamp or carry a flashlight if you're rucking at dawn, dusk, or night. This enhances your visibility and helps you see obstacles.

9. Pack a First Aid Kit

-

- Basic Supplies : Include adhesive bandages, antiseptic wipes, pain relievers, blister treatment, and any personal medications.

-

Emergency Items   : Carry a small multitool, emergency blanket, and a whistle for emergencies.

10. Ruck with a Buddy

-       Safety in Numbers : Rucking with a partner or group can enhance safety and make the experience more enjoyable.

-       Accountability   : A rucking buddy can help keep you motivated and accountable.

11. Monitor Weather Conditions

-       Preparation   : Check the weather forecast before heading out. Dress appropriately and carry necessary gear, such as rain jackets or sun protection.

-       Adaptability   : Be prepared to adjust your plans if weather conditions change unexpectedly.

12. **Understand Your Limits**

Personal Assessment : Know your fitness level and adjust your rucking plans accordingly. Don't attempt overly challenging routes or weights too soon.

-   Gradual Progression : Increase weight and distance gradually to allow your body to adapt and build strength over time.

13. **Stay Connected**

-      Communication : Inform someone of your rucking plans, including your route and expected return time.

-      Mobile Phone : Carry a fully charged mobile phone for emergencies. Consider using a fitness app to track your route and progress.

14. **Incorporate Rest Days**

-

- Recovery : Allow your body time to recover between rucking sessions. Overtraining can lead to injuries and burnout.

Variety : Mix rucking with other forms of exercise to avoid overuse injuries and maintain overall fitness.

15. Learn Basic Navigation

- Maps : Carry a map of your route, especially if you're exploring new areas or trails.

- Navigation Skills : Familiarize yourself with basic navigation skills, such as reading a map and using a compass or GPS device.

16. Emergency Preparedness

- Emergency Plan : Have a plan for emergencies, including knowing the location of the nearest medical facilities and having emergency contact information readily available.

-

-        First Aid Training : Consider taking a basic first aid course to be better prepared for handling injuries or emergencies.

Advanced Safety Tips

For those looking to take their rucking to the next level, consider these advanced safety tips:

1. Increase Weight and Distance Gradually

-       Progressive Overload : Gradually increase the weight and distance of your rucks to continue challenging your body without risking injury.

-       Strength Training   : Incorporate strength training exercises to build the muscles needed for rucking, such as squats, lunges, and deadlifts.

2. Tackle Diverse Terrains

-       Hill Rucking : Once you're comfortable with flat terrain, start incorporating hills into your routes to increase intensity.

-       Trail Rucking : Explore off-road trails for a more challenging and varied rucking experience.

3. Join Organized Rucking Events

-        Rucking Challenges : Participate in rucking events or challenges to test your endurance and connect with the rucking community.

-        Group Rucks : Join group rucking sessions to benefit from shared knowledge, motivation, and safety in numbers.

4. Optimize Your Nutrition

-        Pre-Ruck Nutrition : Eat a balanced meal or snack before rucking to fuel your body. Include carbohydrates, protein, and healthy fats.

-        Post-Ruck Recovery : Refuel after your ruck with a meal or snack that includes protein and carbohydrates to aid muscle recovery.

5. Enhance Your Hydration Strategy

-        Hydration Packs : Consider using a hydration pack or bladder for longer rucks to ensure you have easy access to water.

-        Electrolyte Balance : Use electrolyte tablets or drinks to maintain electrolyte balance, especially during longer or more intense rucks.

6. **Utilize Technology**

-       Fitness Apps : Use fitness apps to track your rucking sessions, monitor progress, and stay motivated.

-       Wearable Devices : Invest in a wearable device, such as a smartwatch or fitness tracker, to monitor your heart rate, distance, and other vital statistics.

Conclusion

Rucking is a highly beneficial and accessible form of exercise, but safety should always be a priority. By following these essential tips, new ruckers can minimize risks and enjoy the numerous benefits that rucking has to offer. Start slow, choose the right gear, maintain proper form, and listen to your body. Stay hydrated, informed, and prepared for emergencies. With careful planning and gradual progression, rucking can be a rewarding and sustainable path to better health and fitness. So gear up, stay safe, and embark on your rucking journey with confidence.

Setting Realistic Goals

Setting Realistic Goals: A Comprehensive Guide

Setting goals is a fundamental step towards achieving success in any area of life, be it personal, professional, or academic. However, the key to attaining these goals lies in making them realistic and achievable. Unrealistic goals can lead to frustration, burnout, and a sense of failure, while realistic goals can motivate, inspire, and provide a clear path to success. This guide will explore the importance of setting realistic goals and provide a step-by-step approach to help you create and achieve them.

The Importance of Setting Realistic Goals

1.   Clarity and Focus : Realistic goals provide a clear direction and focus. They help you understand what you want to achieve and the steps needed to get there.

2.   Motivation   : Achievable goals keep you motivated. As you reach milestones, the sense of accomplishment propels you forward.

3.   Time Management   : Realistic goals enable better time management. They help you prioritize tasks and allocate time effectively.

4.   Resource Allocation   : When goals are realistic, you can better allocate resources, whether they be time, money, or effort.

5.   Stress Reduction : Unrealistic goals can lead to stress and anxiety. Realistic goals reduce these feelings by setting attainable targets.

Step-by-Step Guide to Setting Realistic Goals

1. Self-Assessment and Reflection

-     Identify Your Values : Reflect on what is important to you. Your goals should align with your core values and beliefs.

-     Assess Your Strengths and Weaknesses : Understand your strengths to leverage them and acknowledge your weaknesses to address them.

\-   Define Your Purpose : Consider what you want to achieve and why. Understanding your purpose gives your goals meaning.

2.   SMART Goals Framework

The SMART framework is a popular method for setting realistic goals. SMART stands for Specific, Measurable, Achievable, Relevant, and Timebound.

\-   Specific : Define your goal clearly. Vague goals are hard to achieve. Instead of saying, "I want to get fit," specify, "I want to run a 5K marathon."

\-   Measurable : Establish criteria to track progress. A measurable goal answers questions like "How much?" and "How many?"

\-   Achievable : Ensure your goal is realistic given your current situation and resources. It should stretch your abilities but remain possible.

\-   Relevant : Your goal should matter to you and align with other relevant objectives. It should be worthwhile and pertinent to your long-term plans.

-

Time-bound : Set a deadline. A time-bound goal creates a sense of urgency and helps you stay focused.

3. Break Down Goals into Smaller Steps

Large goals can be overwhelming. Breaking them into smaller, manageable steps makes them more achievable.

- Sub-goals : Divide your main goal into subgoals. For instance, if your goal is to write a book, sub-goals could include writing an outline, completing a chapter, and editing drafts.

- Tasks and Milestones : Identify specific tasks needed to achieve each sub-goal. Set milestones to track your progress and celebrate small wins.

4. Create an Action Plan

An action plan outlines the steps you need to take to reach your goal. It includes timelines, resources needed, and potential obstacles.

-       Timeline : Establish a timeline for each sub-goal and task. This helps keep you on track and ensures steady progress.

-       Resources : Identify the resources you need, such as time, money, tools, and support from others.

-       Obstacles   : Anticipate potential challenges and plan how to overcome them. This proactive approach prevents setbacks from derailing your progress.

5. Monitor Progress and Adjust as Needed

Regularly monitoring your progress keeps you accountable and allows for adjustments if necessary.

-       Tracking Tools   : Use tools like journals, apps, or spreadsheets to track your progress. Documenting your journey provides motivation and insights.

-

- Review and Reflect : Periodically review your progress. Reflect on what is working and what isn't.
Adjust your action plan if needed.

Flexibility : Be flexible and open to change. Life is unpredictable, and sometimes you may need to adjust your goals or timelines.

6. Seek Support and Accountability

Having support and accountability can significantly enhance your chances of success.

- Accountability Partners : Find someone who can hold you accountable. This could be a friend, family member, mentor, or coach.

- Support Systems : Build a support system of people who encourage and assist you. Surround yourself with positive influences.

-       Feedback   :   Seek feedback from others. Constructive criticism can provide valuable insights and help you improve.

7. Celebrate Achievements

Celebrating your achievements, no matter how small, is crucial for maintaining motivation and a positive mindset.

-       Reward Yourself   : Reward yourself when you reach milestones. This can be as simple as treating yourself to something you enjoy.

-       Acknowledge Progress : Acknowledge the progress you've made. Reflect on how far you've come and the effort you've put in.

Examples of Setting Realistic Goals

1. Personal Fitness Goal

-

- Unrealistic Goal : Lose 30 pounds in one month.

- Realistic Goal : Lose 1-2 pounds per week by incorporating regular exercise and a balanced diet.

- Specific : I want to lose 1-2 pounds per week.

- Measurable : Track weight loss progress weekly.

Achievable : Losing 1-2 pounds per week is a healthy and attainable goal.

- Relevant : This goal aligns with my desire to improve my health.

- Time-bound : I aim to lose 10-20 pounds in the next 10 weeks.

2. Professional Development Goal

- Unrealistic Goal : Become the CEO of a company within a year.

- Realistic Goal : Gain a promotion to a managerial position within two years by enhancing skills and performance.

- Specific : I want to be promoted to a managerial position.

- Measurable : Track progress through performance reviews and skill assessments.

- Achievable : Enhancing skills and improving performance within two years is attainable.

- Relevant : This goal aligns with my career aspirations.

- Time-bound : I aim to achieve this promotion within two years.

3. Academic Goal

- Unrealistic Goal : Master a new language fluently in three months.

-

- Realistic Goal   : Achieve conversational proficiency in a new language within one year by studying regularly.

- Specific : I want to achieve conversational proficiency in French.

- Measurable   : Track progress through language assessments and practice conversations.

- Achievable   : Studying regularly and practicing for a year makes this goal attainable.

- Relevant : This goal aligns with my interest in learning a new language.

- Time-bound   : I aim to achieve conversational proficiency within one year.

Overcoming Common Challenges in Goal Setting

1. Procrastination

- Solution : Break tasks into smaller, manageable steps. Set deadlines and create a schedule to stay on track. Use productivity techniques such as the Pomodoro Technique to maintain focus.

2. Lack of Motivation

- Solution : Remind yourself of the reasons behind your goals. Visualize the benefits of achieving them. Surround yourself with supportive and motivating individuals.

3. Fear of Failure

- Solution : Embrace failure as a learning opportunity. Understand that setbacks are part of the journey. Develop a growth mindset and focus on continuous improvement.

4. Inconsistent Progress

-       Solution : Regularly review and adjust your action plan. Stay flexible and adapt to changing circumstances. Celebrate small achievements to maintain momentum.

5. Resource Constraints

-       Solution   : Identify alternative resources or creative solutions. Prioritize tasks and focus on what's essential. Seek support from others to overcome resource limitations.

Maintaining Long-Term Success

1. Continual Learning

-        Growth Mindset   : Adopt a growth mindset, which emphasizes learning and improvement. Stay curious and open to new ideas.

-        Skill Development   : Continuously develop your skills and knowledge. Take courses, attend workshops, and seek mentorship.

2. Adaptability

-        Flexibility : Be willing to adapt your goals and plans as circumstances change. Life is dynamic, and flexibility is key to long-term success.

-        Resilience   : Build resilience by learning from setbacks and persisting through challenges. Focus on solutions rather than problems.

3. Sustainable Practices

-        Balanced Approach   : Maintain a balance between work, rest, and recreation.

Avoid burnout by taking care of your physical and mental well-being.

-	Healthy Habits : Develop healthy habits that support your goals. These may include regular exercise, a balanced diet, adequate sleep, and mindfulness practices.

4. Vision and Purpose

-	Long-Term Vision : Keep your long-term vision and purpose in mind. This provides direction and motivation during challenging times.

-	Alignment : Ensure your goals remain aligned with your values and aspirations. Periodically reassess your goals to stay on the right path.

CHAPTER 4

Mastering Rucking Techniques

The Basics of Rucking

1. Understanding Rucking : Rucking is a versatile workout that can be tailored to different fitness levels and goals. It originated from military training and has since become popular among fitness enthusiasts for its numerous benefits, including improved cardiovascular health, increased strength, and enhanced mental toughness.

2. Benefits of Rucking :

    - Cardiovascular Health : The added weight increases heart rate, improving cardiovascular fitness.

-      Strength Building : Rucking engages multiple muscle groups, including the legs, back, shoulders, and core.

Calorie Burn : The additional effort required to carry the weight leads to higher calorie expenditure.

-	Low Impact : Compared to running, rucking is gentler on the joints.

-	Mental Resilience : The physical challenge of rucking boosts mental toughness and discipline.

Preparing for Rucking

1.	Choosing the Right Gear :

-	Backpack : Invest in a durable, comfortable backpack with padded shoulder straps and a waist belt. Ensure it fits well to avoid strain.

-	Footwear : Wear supportive shoes or boots suitable for walking or hiking. Proper footwear reduces the risk of blisters and injuries.

-	Clothing : Dress in layers to adapt to changing weather conditions. Choose moisture-wicking fabrics to stay dry and comfortable.

2. Selecting the Right Weight :

-        Starting Weight : Beginners should start with a light weight, around 10% of their body weight.

Gradually increase the weight as your strength and endurance improve.

-        Adjustable Weights : Use household items, such as water bottles or books, or invest in weight plates designed for rucking.

3. Warming Up and Cooling Down :

-        Warm-Up : Perform a 5-10 minute warm-up with light stretching or brisk walking to prepare your muscles and joints.

-        Cool Down : After your ruck, cool down with gentle stretching to aid recovery and prevent muscle stiffness.

Mastering Rucking Techniques

1. Proper Posture and Form :

-

    -      Posture : Keep your back straight and shoulders back. Engage your core muscles to maintain stability.

    -      Stride   : Walk with a natural stride, allowing your arms to swing freely. Avoid taking overly long or short steps.

Load Distribution : Ensure the weight in your backpack is evenly distributed to prevent imbalances and reduce strain on your body.

2. Efficient Breathing Techniques :

    -      Rhythmic Breathing   : Practice rhythmic breathing to maintain a steady pace. Inhale deeply through your nose and exhale through your mouth.

    -      Breath Control : Use breath control techniques to manage exertion. Take deep, controlled breaths, especially during uphill climbs or when carrying heavier loads.

3. Pacing and Cadence :

    -      Consistent Pace   : Maintain a consistent pace throughout your ruck. Avoid starting too fast, which can lead to early fatigue.

-        Cadence : Aim for a steady cadence, taking about 120-140 steps per minute. Adjust your pace based on terrain and load.

4.   Navigating Different Terrains :

-

Flat Surfaces : Focus on maintaining a steady pace and proper form. Use flat surfaces to build endurance.

- Uphill Climbs : Shorten your stride and lean slightly forward. Engage your glutes and thighs to power your ascent.

- Downhill Descents : Take shorter steps and maintain control. Lean slightly back to prevent falling forward.

- Uneven Terrain : Watch your step and maintain balance. Use trekking poles for additional stability if needed.

5. Incorporating Strength Training :

- Leg Strength : Perform exercises like squats, lunges, and calf raises to build leg strength.

- Core Strength : Strengthen your core with exercises like planks, Russian twists, and mountain climbers.

- Upper Body Strength : Incorporate push-ups, pull-ups, and shoulder presses to enhance upper body strength.

-

6. Hydration and Nutrition :

    Hydration : Stay hydrated by drinking water before, during, and after your ruck. Use hydration packs or carry water bottles.

       -      Nutrition   : Fuel your body with balanced meals and snacks. Include carbohydrates for energy, protein for muscle repair, and fats for sustained energy.

7. Monitoring Progress :

       -      Tracking Tools : Use fitness apps, journals, or spreadsheets to track your progress. Document your distance, weight, pace, and any challenges.

       -      Regular Assessments : Periodically assess your progress. Adjust your training plan based on your performance and goals.

Advanced Rucking Techniques

1. Interval Training :

-

- High-Intensity Intervals : Incorporate highintensity intervals by alternating between fast-paced rucking and slower recovery periods.

Hill Repeats : Perform hill repeats by rucking up a hill at a fast pace, then walking back down for recovery. Repeat several times.

2. Long-Distance Rucking :

- Building Endurance : Gradually increase your rucking distance over time. Aim to complete longer rucks at a comfortable pace.

- Fueling and Hydration : Plan for longer rucks by carrying sufficient water and nutrition. Take regular breaks to refuel and rehydrate.

3. Rucking with Variable Loads :

- Load Variation : Incorporate variable loads by changing the weight in your backpack. Use lighter loads for endurance training and heavier loads for strength training.

-

- Sandbag Rucking : Use sandbags as an alternative load. Sandbags can shift during the ruck, adding an element of instability and increasing the challenge.

4. Incorporating Other Exercises :

Bodyweight Exercises : Include bodyweight exercises like push-ups, burpees, and squats during your ruck. Stop at regular intervals to perform these exercises.

- Circuit Training : Combine rucking with circuit training. Create circuits that include rucking, strength exercises, and agility drills.

5. Mental Toughness and Resilience :

- Visualization : Practice visualization techniques to prepare mentally for challenging rucks. Visualize yourself completing the ruck successfully.

- Positive Self-Talk : Use positive self-talk to stay motivated and focused. Replace negative thoughts with encouraging affirmations.

-

- Mindfulness : Practice mindfulness during your ruck. Focus on your breathing, surroundings, and sensations to stay present and reduce stress.

Common Rucking Mistakes and How to Avoid Them

1. Overloading Too Soon :

Mistake : Starting with too much weight can lead to injury and burnout.

- Solution : Start with a light weight and gradually increase it as your strength and endurance improve.

2. Improper Footwear :

- Mistake : Wearing unsuitable shoes can cause blisters, discomfort, and injuries.

- Solution : Invest in supportive, comfortable footwear designed for walking or hiking.

3. Poor Posture and Form :

- Mistake : Slouching or leaning forward can strain your back and shoulders.

- Solution : Maintain proper posture and form by keeping your back straight, shoulders back, and core engaged.

4. Inadequate Hydration :

- Mistake : Not drinking enough water can lead to dehydration and decreased performance.

Solution : Stay hydrated by drinking water before, during, and after your ruck. Use hydration packs or carry water bottles.

5. Ignoring Recovery :

- Mistake : Neglecting recovery can lead to overtraining and injuries.

- Solution : Incorporate rest days, stretch regularly, and practice active recovery techniques like foam rolling and light walking.

-

6. Not Listening to Your Body :

> -   Mistake   : Ignoring signs of pain or fatigue can lead to serious injuries.

> -   Solution : Pay attention to your body's signals. Rest and seek medical advice if you experience persistent pain or discomfort.

Conclusion

Mastering rucking techniques involves understanding the fundamentals, preparing properly, and continuously improving your skills and endurance. By focusing on proper posture, efficient breathing, pacing, and strength training, you can enhance your rucking performance and reduce the risk of injury. Incorporate advanced techniques like interval training, long-distance rucking, and mental resilience practices to challenge yourself and achieve your goals. Avoid common mistakes by starting slow, investing in the right gear, and prioritizing recovery and hydration. With dedication and consistent effort, you can master the art of rucking and enjoy its numerous physical and mental benefits.

Proper Posture and Form

1. Posture :

    - Head : Keep your head up and look forward, not down at your feet. This helps maintain a natural alignment of your spine.

    - Shoulders : Keep your shoulders back and relaxed. Avoid hunching or rounding them forward.

    - Back : Maintain a straight back. Avoid arching or excessively rounding your spine.

    - Core : Engage your core muscles to provide stability and support for your back.

2. Arm Swing :

-       Allow your arms to swing naturally at your sides. This helps with balance and momentum.

-       Avoid excessive arm movement, which can waste energy.

3. Stride :

-       Walk with a natural stride, neither too long nor too short.

-       Land softly on your heels and roll through to your toes.

-       Maintain a steady rhythm to conserve energy and avoid unnecessary strain.

4. Load Distribution :

-       Ensure the weight in your backpack is evenly distributed. Pack heavier items closer to your back and lighter items further out.

-       Use a backpack with padded shoulder straps and a waist belt to distribute the weight evenly and reduce strain on your shoulders and back.

Efficient Breathing Techniques

1. Rhythmic Breathing :

    -    Practice rhythmic breathing to maintain a steady pace. Inhale deeply through your nose and exhale through your mouth.

    -    Synchronize your breathing with your steps. For example, inhale for three steps and exhale for two steps.

2. Deep Breathing :

    -    Take deep breaths to fully oxygenate your muscles. Shallow breathing can lead to fatigue and decreased performance.

    -    Focus on expanding your diaphragm rather than just your chest.

3. Breath Control :

\-   Use breath control techniques to manage exertion, especially during challenging sections like uphill climbs.

\-   Practice breathing exercises outside of your rucking sessions to improve lung capacity and control.

Pacing and Cadence

1. Consistent Pace :

    \-   Maintain a consistent pace throughout your ruck. Avoid starting too fast, which can lead to early fatigue.

    \-   Find a sustainable speed that allows you to complete your ruck without burning out.

2. Cadence :

    \-   Aim for a steady cadence, typically around 120140 steps per minute.

    \-   Use a metronome or music with a specific beatsper-minute (BPM) to help maintain a consistent cadence.

3. Adjusting Pace :

-        Adjust your pace based on terrain, weather, and load. Slow down on challenging sections and increase speed on easier parts.

-        Listen to your body and avoid pushing too hard if you feel fatigued.

Navigating Different Terrains

1. Flat Surfaces :

-        Focus on maintaining a steady pace and proper form.

-        Use flat surfaces to build endurance and establish a rhythm.

2. Uphill Climbs :

-        Shorten your stride and lean slightly forward from the hips.

-        Engage your glutes and thighs to power your ascent.

-        Use trekking poles for additional support and balance.

3.   Downhill Descents :

-        Take shorter steps and maintain control. Avoid leaning too far back.

-        Use your core and legs to absorb the impact and maintain balance.

-        Use trekking poles to help distribute weight and reduce strain on your knees.

4.   Uneven Terrain :

-        Watch your step and maintain balance. Be mindful of obstacles like rocks, roots, and loose gravel.

-        Use a wider stance for stability and keep your center of gravity low.

-        Trekking poles can provide additional support and help navigate tricky sections.

Incorporating Strength Training

1.   Leg Strength :

-        Perform exercises like squats, lunges, and calf raises to build leg strength.

-        Strong legs help you handle the added weight and reduce fatigue.

2. Core Strength :

-        Strengthen your core with exercises like planks, Russian twists, and mountain climbers.

-        A strong core provides stability and reduces the risk of back injuries.

3. Upper Body Strength :

-        Incorporate push-ups, pull-ups, and shoulder presses to enhance upper body strength.

-        Strong shoulders and back muscles help you carry the load more comfortably.

4. Functional Training :

-        Include functional exercises that mimic the movements you'll encounter while rucking. For example, weighted step-ups and farmer's walks.

-        Train with the same gear and weight you'll use during your ruck to prepare your body for the demands.

Hydration and Nutrition

1. Hydration :

    -        Stay hydrated by drinking water before, during, and after your ruck. Use hydration packs or carry water bottles.

    -        Monitor your urine color to ensure you're adequately hydrated. Aim for a pale yellow color.

2. Electrolyte Balance :

    -        Consume electrolyte-rich drinks or supplements to maintain electrolyte balance, especially during long or intense rucks.

    -        Electrolytes help prevent cramps and maintain proper muscle function.

3. Nutrition :

-       Fuel your body with balanced meals and snacks. Include carbohydrates for energy, protein for muscle repair, and fats for sustained energy.

-       Eat a meal or snack 1-2 hours before your ruck to ensure you have enough energy. Post-ruck, consume protein and carbs to aid recovery.

4. Portable Snacks :

-       Carry portable, nutrient-dense snacks like energy bars, nuts, dried fruit, and jerky.

-       Avoid sugary snacks that can cause energy spikes and crashes.

Interval Training

1. High-Intensity Intervals :

-       Incorporate high-intensity intervals by alternating between fast-paced rucking and slower recovery periods.

-       For example, ruck at a fast pace for 2 minutes, followed by 3 minutes of moderate pace. Repeat for the duration of your workout.

2. Hill Repeats :

-       Perform hill repeats by rucking up a hill at a fast pace, then walking back down for recovery. Repeat several times.

-       Hill repeats improve cardiovascular fitness, leg strength, and endurance.

3. Variable Load Intervals :

-       Alternate between carrying different loads. For example, ruck with a heavy load for 5 minutes, then switch to a lighter load for 10 minutes.

-       This technique challenges your muscles and improves overall strength and endurance.

4. Timed Intervals :

-       Use a timer to structure your interval training. For example, 30 seconds of fast-paced rucking followed by 1 minute of recovery.

-       Gradually increase the intensity and duration of the high-intensity intervals as your fitness improves.

Monitoring Progress

1. Tracking Tools :

    - Use fitness apps, journals, or spreadsheets to track your progress. Document your distance, weight, pace, and any challenges.

    - Review your data regularly to identify patterns and areas for improvement.

2. Regular Assessments :

    - Periodically assess your progress by completing a benchmark ruck. Use the same route, weight, and pace to compare performance over time.

    - Set specific, measurable goals to work towards and celebrate your achievements.

3. Adjusting Goals :

    - Adjust your goals based on your progress and changing circumstances. Be flexible and open to modifying your training plan.

-       Set short-term and long-term goals to keep yourself motivated and focused.

4.   Seeking Feedback :

-       Seek feedback from experienced ruckers or trainers. They can provide valuable insights and advice to help you improve.

-       Join rucking communities or groups to share experiences and learn from others.

Advanced Rucking Techniques

1.   Long-Distance Rucking :

-       Gradually increase your rucking distance over time. Aim to complete longer rucks at a comfortable pace.

-       Plan for longer rucks by carrying sufficient water and nutrition. Take regular breaks to refuel and rehydrate.

2.   Rucking with Variable Loads :

-       Incorporate variable loads by changing the weight in your backpack. Use lighter loads for endurance training and heavier loads for strength training.

-        Sandbags can add an element of instability and increase the challenge.

3. Incorporating Other Exercises :

-        Include bodyweight exercises like push-ups, burpees, and squats during your ruck. Stop at regular intervals to perform these exercises.

-        Combine rucking with circuit training. Create circuits that include rucking, strength exercises, and agility drills.

4. Mental Toughness and Resilience :

-        Practice visualization techniques to prepare mentally for challenging rucks. Visualize yourself completing the ruck successfully.

-        Use positive self-talk to stay motivated and focused. Replace negative thoughts with encouraging affirmations.

-        Practice mindfulness during your ruck. Focus on your breathing, surroundings, and sensations to stay present and reduce stress.

ESSENTIAL RUCKING TECHNIQUE

Maintain a straight spine and a high head. Maintain an upright posture, open your chest, and assume a "proud" stance as you stand tall.

When walking, maintain your upright posture and fully extend your hips.

Stride less than usual, attempting to maintain your foot strike (ground contact) nearer your hips (think minimalist and barefoot jogging).

To avoid long-term knee damage, take flat feet steps and aim for a midfoot to forefoot strike (as in minimalist and barefoot running).

Instead of "pounding," use a "glide stride" to maintain your forward movement, protect your knees, and make sure one foot is always on the ground.

In order to completely "drive the hips," or force the body forward, engage your glutes to provide strength and power to the exercise.

Maintain the shoulders "activated" by pulling them down and back into a somewhat neutral position. If you must shrug to support the weight, think about reducing the amount of weight you're carrying.

Retain a "hollow" or neutrally engaged core, supporting the spine with your lower back and abs.

Keep your posture straight and "stand tall" by keeping your head up, chest open and "proud," and your core engaged. This method prevents usage injuries, engages your muscles in their natural position, and reinforces healthy posture. You're rucking too heavy for your level if you can't do this.

Wait to ruck until you've completed the same distance on foot, or at the very least, walk with 5 pounds less than your desired ruck weight.

Never run with your ruck on; always keep one foot planted firmly on the ground.

To determine the intensity of your workout, use your heart rate (180 – your age as the goal BPM). Walk more quickly to elevate your heart rate.

If you're new to rucking, start with 15–25 pounds, and as a general rule, don't go over 10% of your body weight for smaller and less experienced people.

ADVICE FOR ACCURATE RUCKING

Lean back, keep your head up, and keep your chest open.

Keep your core engaged but neutral.

Reduce the length of your steps.

Avoid running when carrying weight.

Drive the motions with your glutes flexed and your body at full or almost full extension on the

To prevent the weights from moving, pack them high and steadily onto your back.

Select athletic footwear with a moderate amount of cushioning (not too much).

Give up wearing military boots with the high top and ankle support to promote the growth of your lower limbs.

Perfecting Your Posture and Form

Perfecting Your Posture and Form for Rucking

Rucking, a fitness activity involving walking or hiking with a weighted backpack, offers an effective way to improve strength, endurance, and cardiovascular health. To maximize benefits and minimize the risk of injury, it is crucial to maintain proper posture and form. This comprehensive guide will help you perfect your posture and form for rucking, ensuring you get the most out of your workouts.

Importance of Proper Posture and Form

1. Injury Prevention :

-

Proper posture reduces the risk of strains, sprains, and other injuries by ensuring your body moves efficiently and safely.

- Good form helps distribute the weight evenly, minimizing the stress on any single muscle group or joint.

2. Enhanced Performance :

- Maintaining correct posture and form allows you to move more efficiently, conserving energy and improving endurance.

- Efficient movement patterns help you ruck longer distances with less fatigue.

3. Muscle Engagement :

- Proper form ensures that the right muscles are engaged, leading to balanced muscle development.

- It helps target the core, legs, and back muscles effectively, enhancing overall strength.

Key Components of Proper Rucking Posture

-

1.   Head Position :

   Keep your head up and look forward, not down at your feet. This helps maintain a natural alignment of your spine.

   -        Avoid tilting your head forward, which can strain your neck and upper back muscles.

2.   Shoulders and Upper Back :

   -        Keep your shoulders back and relaxed. Avoid hunching or rounding them forward.

   -        Engage your upper back muscles to help stabilize your shoulders and prevent slouching.

3.   Back and Core :

   -        Maintain a straight back. Avoid arching or excessively rounding your spine.

   -        Engage your core muscles to provide stability and support for your back. Think of pulling your belly button towards your spine.

-

4. Hips and Pelvis :

-        Keep your hips level and avoid tilting them forward or backward.

Your pelvis should be in a neutral position to maintain a natural alignment of your spine.

5. Legs and Stride :

-        Walk with a natural stride, neither too long nor too short. Avoid overstriding, which can put unnecessary strain on your muscles and joints.

-        Land softly on your heels and roll through to your toes. Push off with your toes to propel yourself forward.

6. Feet :

-        Keep your feet pointed forward and avoid excessive outward or inward rotation.

-        Distribute your weight evenly across your feet to maintain balance and stability.

-

7. Arms and Hands :

-       Allow your arms to swing naturally at your sides. This helps with balance and momentum.

-       Keep your elbows slightly bent and avoid excessive arm movement, which can waste energy.

Tips for Maintaining Proper Form While Rucking

1. Start with a Light Load :

-   Begin with a lighter weight, around 10% of your body weight, to get used to carrying a load while maintaining proper form.

-   Gradually increase the weight as your strength and endurance improve.

2. Use a Well-Fitted Backpack :

-   Invest in a backpack with padded shoulder straps and a waist belt to distribute the weight evenly and reduce strain on your shoulders and back.

-   Ensure the backpack fits snugly and doesn't shift during your ruck.

3. Adjust the Load Distribution :

-   Pack heavier items closer to your back and lighter items further out to maintain balance and stability.

-        Ensure the weight is evenly distributed to prevent imbalances and reduce strain on your body.

4. Warm-Up and Cool Down :

-        Perform a 5-10 minute warm-up with light stretching or brisk walking to prepare your muscles and joints.

-        After your ruck, cool down with gentle stretching to aid recovery and prevent muscle stiffness.

5. Monitor Your Form Regularly :

-        Periodically check your posture and form during your ruck. Make adjustments as needed to maintain proper alignment.

-        Use reflective surfaces, such as windows or mirrors, or ask a training partner to observe your form.

6. Strengthen Core Muscles :

-        Incorporate core-strengthening exercises, such as planks, Russian twists, and mountain climbers, into your fitness routine.

-

- A strong core provides stability and support, making it easier to maintain proper posture.

7. Focus on Breathing :

Practice rhythmic breathing to maintain a steady pace and reduce tension in your upper body.

- Inhale deeply through your nose and exhale through your mouth, synchronizing your breathing with your steps.

8. Listen to Your Body :

- Pay attention to any signs of discomfort or pain. Adjust your form or reduce the load if you experience persistent issues.

- Rest and seek medical advice if you experience persistent pain or discomfort.

Common Posture Mistakes and How to Correct Them

1. Forward Head Tilt :

-        Mistake   : Tilting your head forward, which strains the neck and upper back muscles.

-        Correction : Keep your head up and look forward. Imagine a string pulling your head upwards to maintain a neutral position.

2. Hunched Shoulders :

-        Mistake   : Rounding your shoulders forward, which can lead to upper back and shoulder pain.

-        Correction : Keep your shoulders back and relaxed. Engage your upper back muscles and open your chest.

3. Excessive Arching or Rounding of the Back :

-        Mistake : Arching your back too much or rounding it excessively, leading to back strain.

-        Correction : Maintain a straight back with a neutral spine. Engage your core to support your back.

4. Overstriding :

-

- Mistake : Taking overly long steps, which can strain your muscles and joints.

- Correction : Walk with a natural stride. Land softly on your heels and roll through to your toes.

5. Poor Load Distribution :

- Mistake : Packing the backpack unevenly, leading to imbalances and strain.

Correction : Pack heavier items closer to your back and lighter items further out. Ensure the weight is evenly distributed.

Advanced Tips for Perfecting Your Form

1. Engage Your Glutes and Hamstrings :

- Focus on engaging your glutes and hamstrings to power your stride. This helps reduce strain on your lower back and improves overall stability.

2. Use Trekking Poles :

-    Consider using trekking poles for additional support and balance, especially on uneven terrain or during long rucks.

-    Trekking poles can help distribute the load more evenly and reduce strain on your knees and lower back.

3. Incorporate Mobility Work :

-    Include mobility exercises, such as hip flexor stretches and thoracic spine rotations, in your fitness routine to improve flexibility and range of motion.

-

Improved mobility helps maintain proper form and reduces the risk of injuries.

4. Mindfulness and Body Awareness :

-       Practice mindfulness during your ruck. Focus on your breathing, surroundings, and sensations to stay present and reduce stress.

-       Pay attention to your body's signals. If you notice discomfort or fatigue, adjust your form or take a break.

5. Footwear Considerations :

-       Wear well-fitted, supportive shoes designed for rucking or hiking. Proper footwear provides stability and reduces the risk of blisters and foot pain.

-       Replace your shoes regularly to ensure they provide adequate support and cushioning.

6. Rucking with Variable Loads :

-       Incorporate variable loads by changing the weight in your backpack. Use lighter loads for endurance training and heavier loads for strength training.

Gradually increase the weight to challenge your muscles and improve overall strength.

7. Interval Training :

-       Include interval training in your rucking routine to build endurance and strength. Alternate between fast-paced rucking and slower recovery periods.

-       For example, ruck at a fast pace for 2 minutes, followed by 3 minutes of moderate pace. Repeat for the duration of your workout.

Incorporating Strength Training

1. Leg Strength :

-       Perform exercises like squats, lunges, and calf raises to build leg strength. Strong legs help you handle the added weight and reduce fatigue.

-

2. Core Strength :

-       Strengthen your core with exercises like planks, Russian twists, and mountain climbers. A strong core provides stability and reduces the risk of back injuries.

3. Upper Body Strength :

-       Incorporate push-ups, pull-ups, and shoulder presses to enhance upper body strength. Strong shoulders and back muscles help you carry the load more comfortably.

4. Functional Training :

-       Include functional exercises that mimic the movements you'll encounter while rucking. For example, weighted step-ups and farmer's walks.

-       Train with the same gear and weight you'll use during your ruck to prepare your body for the demands.

Hydration and Nutrition

1. Hydration :

-       Stay hydrated by drinking water before, during, and after your ruck. Use hydration packs or carry water bottles. Monitor your urine color to ensure you're adequately hydrated. Aim for a pale yellow color.

2. Electrolyte Balance :

   - Consume electrolyte-rich drinks or supplements to maintain electrolyte balance, especially during long or intense rucks. Electrolytes help prevent cramps and maintain proper muscle function.

3. Nutrition :

   - Fuel your body with balanced meals and snacks. Include carbohydrates for energy, protein for muscle repair, and fats for sustained energy. Eat a meal or snack 1-2 hours before your ruck to ensure you have enough energy. Post-ruck, consume protein and carbs to aid recovery.

Interval Training and Pacing

1. Interval Training :

   - Incorporate interval training to build endurance and strength. Alternate between fast-paced rucking and slower recovery periods.

-	For example, ruck at a fast pace for 2 minutes, followed by 3 minutes of moderate pace. Repeat for the duration of your workout.

2.	Pacing :

-	Find a sustainable pace that allows you to maintain proper form and avoid fatigue. Gradually increase your pace as your fitness improves.

Monitoring Progress and Mastering Rucking Techniques

1.	Track Your Progress :

-	Use a fitness tracker or app to monitor your distance, pace, and elevation gain. Keep a training log to track your progress and set goals.

2.	Set Realistic Goals :

-	Set achievable goals based on your fitness level and gradually increase the intensity and duration of your rucks.

3. Mastering Techniques :

-       Practice different rucking techniques, such as uphill and downhill rucking, to prepare for various terrains. Join a rucking group or find a training partner for motivation and support.

Increasing Weight and Distance Safely

Why Increase Weight and Distance?

1. Strength Development :

-       Heavier weights challenge your muscles, promoting growth and increasing overall strength.

2. Endurance Building :

-       Longer distances improve cardiovascular health and stamina, allowing you to sustain physical activity for extended periods.

3. Enhanced Calorie Burn :

    -       Increasing both weight and distance elevates the intensity of your workouts, leading to higher calorie expenditure.

4. Preparation for Advanced Challenges :

    -       Gradually increasing weight and distance prepares you for more demanding rucking events and activities, such as military training or rucking competitions.

Steps to Safely Increase Weight and Distance

1. Assess Your Current Fitness Level :

    -       Before increasing weight or distance, evaluate your current fitness level. Ensure that you can comfortably complete your current rucks without excessive fatigue or discomfort.

-        Track your current distance, weight, and time to set a baseline.

2. Incremental Increases :

-        Weight : Increase the weight in your backpack by small increments, typically 5-10% of the current weight, every 2-4 weeks. This gradual increase allows your body to adapt without overwhelming it.

-        Distance : Add distance incrementally, generally by 0.5 to 1 mile every 1-2 weeks, depending on your current distance and fitness level.

3. Listen to Your Body :

-        Pay close attention to how your body responds to increased weight and distance. If you experience pain (beyond typical muscle soreness) or excessive fatigue, reduce the weight or distance and allow for more recovery time.

4. Maintain Proper Form :

-        As you increase weight and distance, maintaining proper posture and form becomes even more critical to prevent injuries.

\-   Ensure your backpack is well-fitted, and the weight is evenly distributed.

5. Strength Training :

\-   Incorporate strength training exercises into your routine to build the muscles needed for rucking.

Focus on core, leg, and back exercises to support the increased load.

6. Flexibility and Mobility Work :

\-   Regularly perform stretching and mobility exercises to maintain flexibility and prevent stiffness and injuries.

Detailed Process for Increasing Weight

1. Initial Weight Assessment :

\-   Start with a weight that is 10-15% of your body weight if you are new to rucking. For those more experienced, begin with a comfortable weight that does not cause strain.

2. Add Weight Gradually :

-       Increase the weight by 5-10% every 2-4 weeks. For example, if you start with a 20-pound backpack, add 1-2 pounds after a few weeks.

-       Use weight plates, sandbags, or other compact weight options to ensure the added weight is evenly distributed in your pack.

3. Monitor and Adjust :

-       Keep a training log to track the weight you carry and your body's response. Note any discomfort or pain and adjust accordingly.

4. Recovery and Rest :

-       Allow adequate recovery between rucking sessions, especially when increasing weight. Rest days are essential for muscle recovery and preventing overuse injuries.

Detailed Process for Increasing Distance

1. Baseline Distance :

-       Determine your current comfortable rucking distance. This is the distance you can cover without significant fatigue or soreness.

2. Incremental Distance Increase :

-       Increase your distance by 0.5 to 1 mile every 1-2 weeks. For example, if you comfortably ruck 3 miles, aim for 3.5 to 4 miles after a couple of weeks.

-

Ensure that each new distance feels manageable before further increasing it.

3. Monitor Your Pacing :

    -       Maintain a steady pace that allows you to complete the increased distance without undue strain. Focus on consistent pacing rather than speed.

4. Endurance Training :

    -       Incorporate endurance training into your routine, such as longer, slower rucks to build cardiovascular fitness and stamina.

5. Cross-Training :

    -       Engage in cross-training activities, such as swimming, cycling, or running, to improve overall endurance and give your rucking muscles a break.

Combining Weight and Distance Increases

1. Sequential Increases :

Avoid increasing both weight and distance simultaneously. Focus on one aspect at a time to prevent overwhelming your body.

-    For example, increase weight for a few weeks while maintaining the same distance, then focus on increasing distance while keeping the weight constant.

2. Balanced Progression :

-    Once you have successfully increased weight and distance independently, you can start to combine them gradually. For instance, increase your weight slightly while also adding a small distance increment.

3. Periodization :

-    Use a periodization approach where you cycle through phases of increasing weight, increasing distance, and recovery. This helps prevent burnout and ensures continuous improvement.

Safety Tips and Best Practices

1. Hydration and Nutrition :

Stay hydrated and fuel your body properly. Carry enough water and high-energy snacks to sustain your longer, heavier rucks.

2. Gear Considerations :

-   Ensure your backpack has good support, with padded straps and a waist belt to distribute weight effectively.

-   Wear appropriate footwear that provides good support and cushioning for the increased load and distance.

3. Warm-Up and Cool Down :

-   Always warm up before your rucks with dynamic stretches or light walking to prepare your muscles.

-   Cool down with static stretches to enhance recovery and flexibility.

-

4. Use a Training Plan :

-        Follow a structured training plan that gradually increases weight and distance. This helps maintain a consistent progression and prevents overtraining.

5. Seek Professional Advice :

    -       Consider consulting with a fitness trainer or physical therapist, especially if you are new to rucking or have pre-existing conditions. They can provide personalized advice and help design a safe progression plan.

    Monitoring Progress

1. Keep a Training Log :

    -       Record your rucking sessions, including weight, distance, time, and any physical responses. This helps track progress and identify patterns.

2. Set Achievable Goals :

    -       Set realistic short-term and long-term goals based on your current fitness level and desired outcomes. Adjust your plan as needed to stay on track.

3. Celebrate Milestones :

-	Recognize and celebrate your progress. Achieving milestones, such as a new distance or weight goal, helps maintain motivation and commitment.

Troubleshooting Common Rucking Challenges

Troubleshooting Common Rucking Challenges and What You Can Do

Rucking, which involves walking or hiking with a weighted backpack, is an excellent way to build strength, endurance, and cardiovascular fitness. However, as with any physical activity, rucking can present various challenges. Understanding these common issues and knowing how to address them can help you maintain an effective and enjoyable rucking routine. This guide explores typical rucking challenges and provides solutions to overcome them.

1. Blisters

Problem : Blisters are a common issue, especially for those new to rucking or increasing their distance and weight.

Solutions :

- Proper Footwear : Invest in high-quality, wellfitting shoes designed for hiking or rucking. Ensure they provide adequate support and cushioning.

- Socks : Wear moisture-wicking, seamless socks to reduce friction and keep your feet dry. Consider double-layer socks for additional protection.

- Lubricants : Apply anti-chafing balms or petroleum jelly to areas prone to blisters before rucking.

- Break-In Period : Gradually break in new shoes by wearing them for short rucks before attempting longer distances.

- Foot Care : Keep your feet clean and dry. If you feel a hot spot developing, stop and apply a blister pad or moleskin to prevent further friction.

2. Back Pain

Problem : Carrying a heavy backpack can lead to back pain, especially if your form is incorrect.

Solutions :

- Proper Posture : Maintain a straight back, engage your core, and avoid leaning forward or backward excessively.

- Backpack Fit : Ensure your backpack fits snugly and distribute the weight evenly. Use the waist and chest straps to reduce the load on your shoulders.

- Weight Distribution : Pack heavier items closer to your back and lighter items farther away to maintain balance.

- Strength Training : Incorporate exercises that strengthen your back and core muscles, such as planks, deadlifts, and rows.

- Gradual Increases : Increase the weight of your backpack gradually to allow your body to adapt.

3. Shoulder and Neck Pain

Problem : Strain on the shoulders and neck from carrying a weighted backpack can cause discomfort and pain.

Solutions :

-

Adjust Straps : Make sure your backpack's shoulder straps are well-padded and adjusted to distribute weight evenly.

-       Load Management : Avoid overloading your backpack. Stick to weight increments that your body can handle comfortably.

-       Stretching : Perform shoulder and neck stretches before and after your ruck to maintain flexibility and reduce tension.

-       Strength Training : Strengthen your shoulder and neck muscles with exercises like shoulder presses, shrugs, and resistance band exercises.

4. Knee Pain

Problem : Knee pain can result from the added weight and impact of rucking, especially on uneven terrain or inclines.

Solutions :

-

- Footwear : Wear shoes with good arch support and cushioning to absorb shock and reduce knee strain.

Proper Form : Maintain good posture and avoid locking your knees. Keep a slight bend to absorb impact.

- Strengthening Exercises : Strengthen the muscles around your knees, such as quadriceps, hamstrings, and calves, with exercises like squats, lunges, and leg presses.

- Gradual Progression : Increase your distance and weight gradually to give your knees time to adapt.

5. Dehydration

Problem : Rucking can lead to dehydration, especially in hot or humid conditions.

Solutions :

-

-        Hydration Plan : Drink water regularly before, during, and after your ruck. Aim to consume about 16-20 ounces of water every hour during your ruck.

-        Electrolytes : Consider drinking electrolyte solutions or sports drinks to replace lost minerals and maintain hydration balance.

Hydration Packs : Use hydration packs or carry water bottles in your backpack for easy access to fluids.

6. Overheating

Problem   : Rucking in hot weather can cause overheating, leading to heat exhaustion or heat stroke.

Solutions :

-        Clothing : Wear lightweight, breathable, and moisture-wicking clothing to help regulate your body temperature.

-        Timing : Ruck during cooler parts of the day, such as early morning or late evening.

-

-        Shade and Rest : Take breaks in shaded areas to cool down and drink water. Listen to your body and rest if you feel overheated.

-        Cooling Aids   : Use cooling towels or bandanas around your neck to help reduce your body temperature.

7. Lack of Motivation

Problem : Maintaining motivation for regular rucking can be challenging, especially when progress seems slow.

Solutions :

-       Set Goals : Establish short-term and long-term rucking goals to keep you focused and motivated.

-       Track Progress : Use a fitness tracker or app to monitor your progress and celebrate milestones.

-       Join a Group : Ruck with a group or find a rucking buddy for social support and accountability.

-       Vary Routes : Change your rucking routes to keep things interesting and explore new areas.

-       Incorporate Challenges : Participate in rucking events or virtual challenges to add excitement and a sense of accomplishment.

8. Time Management

Problem : Finding time for regular rucking sessions can be difficult with a busy schedule.

Solutions :

-        Plan Ahead : Schedule your rucking sessions in advance and treat them as important appointments.

-        Combine Activities : Incorporate rucking into your daily routine, such as walking to work or running errands with your backpack.

-        Shorter Sessions : If time is limited, opt for shorter, more frequent rucking sessions instead of long ones.

-        Family Involvement : Involve family members in your rucking activities to spend time together while staying active.

9. Plateaus in Progress

Problem : Hitting a plateau in your rucking progress can be frustrating and demotivating.

Solutions :

-       Change Variables : Vary the weight, distance, terrain, and pace of your rucks to challenge your body in new ways.

-       Cross-Training : Incorporate other forms of exercise, such as running, cycling, or swimming, to improve overall fitness and break through plateaus.

-       Interval Training : Add intervals of faster walking or jogging to your rucks to increase intensity and boost endurance.

-       Strength Training : Focus on building strength through targeted exercises to enhance your rucking performance.

CHAPTER 5

Building Your Rucking Routine

Building Your Rucking Routine: What You Can Do

Rucking, the activity of walking or hiking with a weighted backpack, is an excellent way to build strength, endurance, and cardiovascular fitness. Establishing a well-structured rucking routine is essential for maximizing the benefits of this activity while minimizing the risk of injury. This guide will help you design a balanced rucking routine, including tips on frequency, intensity, and variety to ensure continuous progress and enjoyment.

Understanding the Basics of Rucking

Before diving into routine building, it's essential to understand the fundamental components of rucking:

1.   Weight : The weight in your backpack can vary based on your fitness level and goals.

Beginners should start with 10-15% of their body weight.

2.   Distance : The distance you cover can range from short walks of 1-2 miles to long hikes of 10+ miles, depending on your experience and goals.

3.   Terrain : Rucking can be done on various terrains, from flat sidewalks to rugged trails, each providing different challenges and benefits.

4.   Pace : Your walking speed will affect the intensity of your workout. A faster pace will increase cardiovascular benefits, while a slower pace with more weight focuses on strength building.

Setting Goals for Your Rucking Routine

Setting clear and achievable goals is the first step in building an effective rucking routine. Your goals will determine the specifics of your routine:

1.   Fitness Goals : Are you aiming to improve overall fitness, lose weight, build strength, or train for an event?

2.   Frequency Goals : How often do you plan to ruck each week? Most people find that 3-4 times per week is manageable and effective.

3.   Progression Goals : How will you increase the weight and distance over time to continue challenging your body and making progress?

Structuring Your Weekly Rucking Routine

A well-rounded rucking routine should include a mix of rucking sessions, strength training, rest, and recovery. Here's a sample weekly structure:

1. Day 1: Short Ruck (Low Weight)

    - Goal   : Warm-up and maintain basic conditioning.

    - Details : 1-2 miles with a light pack (10% of body weight), on flat terrain, at a moderate pace.

2. Day 2: Strength Training

    - Goal   : Build muscle strength to support rucking.

    - Details : Focus on core, legs, and back exercises like squats, lunges, deadlifts, and planks.

3. Day 3: Medium Ruck (Moderate Weight)

   - Goal   : Increase endurance and build strength.

   - Details : 3-4 miles with a moderate pack (15% of body weight), on varied terrain, at a steady pace.

4. Day 4: Rest or Active Recovery

   - Goal : Allow your muscles to recover and prevent overuse injuries.

   - Details : Rest completely or engage in light activities like stretching, yoga, or a casual walk.

5. Day 5: Interval Ruck (Moderate Weight)

   - Goal : Improve cardiovascular fitness and stamina.

   - Details : 2-3 miles with a moderate pack, alternating between fast and slow paces or adding hill intervals.

6. Day 6: Strength Training

- Goal : Continue building muscle strength.

- Details : Similar to Day 2, with a focus on different muscle groups to ensure balanced strength development.

7. Day 7: Long Ruck (Higher Weight)

- Goal   : Build endurance and simulate longer, more demanding rucks.

- Details : 5-7 miles with a heavier pack (20% of body weight), on varied terrain, at a steady pace.

Progression and Adaptation

To continue making progress and avoid plateaus, you need to gradually increase the weight and distance in your rucking routine. Here are some tips:

1.   Incremental Increases : Increase the weight in your pack by 5-10% every few weeks. Similarly, add 0.5 to 1 mile to your rucking distance every few weeks.

2.   Variety : Change up your routes, terrains, and paces to challenge your body in different ways. This also keeps your routine interesting and engaging.

3.   Listen to Your Body : Pay attention to signs of fatigue or discomfort. Adjust your routine as needed to prevent overtraining and injuries.

Incorporating Other Forms of Exercise

While rucking is highly effective, incorporating other forms of exercise can enhance your overall fitness and prevent overuse injuries:

1.   Cross-Training   : Activities like cycling, swimming, or running can improve cardiovascular fitness and give your rucking muscles a break.

2.   Flexibility and Mobility : Regular stretching, yoga, or mobility exercises can improve flexibility, reduce muscle tightness, and prevent injuries.

3.   Balance and Stability : Exercises like balance drills, single-leg stands, and stability ball workouts can enhance your balance and stability, which are crucial for rucking on varied terrains.

Nutrition and Hydration

Proper nutrition and hydration are essential components of any fitness routine, including rucking:

1.   Pre-Ruck Fueling : Eat a balanced meal with carbohydrates, protein, and healthy fats 2-3 hours before rucking. Consider a light snack if you're rucking in the early morning.

2.   Hydration : Drink water before, during, and after your ruck. Carry a hydration pack or water bottles in your backpack for easy access.

3.   Post-Ruck Recovery : Consume a meal or snack with protein and carbohydrates within an hour of finishing your ruck to aid muscle recovery.

Tracking Your Progress

Keeping track of your rucking sessions helps you monitor your progress and make necessary adjustments:

1.   Training Log : Record the details of each ruck, including distance, weight, time, terrain, and

how you felt. This helps you identify patterns and make informed changes.

2.   Fitness Apps : Use fitness tracking apps to log your rucks, set goals, and track progress over time. Many apps also provide insights and tips to improve your performance.

3.   Regular Assessments : Periodically assess your fitness level, including strength, endurance, and body composition. This helps you stay motivated and adjust your routine as needed.

Staying Motivated

Maintaining motivation is crucial for long-term success. Here are some tips to stay motivated:

1.   Set Clear Goals : Define specific, achievable goals for your rucking routine. Break them down into short-term and long-term objectives.

2.   Find a Rucking Community : Join local rucking groups or online communities to connect with likeminded individuals, share experiences, and participate in group rucks.

3.   Challenge Yourself : Sign up for rucking events, virtual challenges, or charity rucks to add excitement and purpose to your routine.

4.   Celebrate Milestones : Recognize and celebrate your achievements, whether it's completing a longer distance, increasing weight, or hitting a new personal best.

Beginner's Guide: First Steps to Rucking

Choosing Your Gear

Backpack :

Your backpack is your most critical piece of equipment. Look for a durable, comfortable backpack with padded shoulder straps and a waist belt to distribute the weight evenly. The pack should fit snugly to prevent shifting and discomfort during your ruck. Backpacks specifically designed for rucking often come with additional features like reinforced stitching and hydration bladder compatibility.

Weights :

Start with a weight that is 10-15% of your body weight. Common weights include weight plates, sandbags, or even water bottles. As you become more comfortable, you can gradually increase the weight. Make sure the weights are securely packed to prevent movement within the backpack.

Footwear :

Invest in a good pair of walking or hiking shoes. Look for shoes that offer excellent support, cushioning, and a good grip. Proper footwear will help prevent blisters and foot pain, making your rucking experience more enjoyable.

Clothing :

Wear moisture-wicking, breathable clothing to keep you comfortable during your rucks. Layer appropriately for the weather, and consider wearing a hat and sunscreen for sun protection.

Basic Technique

Posture :

Maintain a tall posture with your shoulders back, core engaged, and head up. Avoid leaning forward or backward excessively, as this can cause strain on your back and shoulders.

Walking Form :

Walk with a natural stride, keeping your steps steady and smooth. Swing your arms naturally for balance and rhythm. Ensure your feet land heel to toe to distribute impact evenly.

Breathing :

Maintain a steady breathing pattern. Breathe deeply and evenly to ensure adequate oxygen intake. This will help you maintain your energy levels throughout your ruck.

Starting Routine

Duration :

Begin with short rucks of 20-30 minutes. This will help you get used to carrying the weight and walking with proper form.

Frequency :

Aim for 2-3 times per week. This frequency allows your body to adapt to the new exercise while providing enough recovery time.

Progression :

Gradually increase the weight and duration of your rucks. Aim to add weight incrementally and extend your rucks by 5-10 minutes every couple of weeks. Listen to your body and adjust your progression based on how you feel.

Safety Tips

Warm-Up and Cool-Down :

Perform a light warm-up before starting and cool down with stretching afterward. This helps prepare your muscles for the workout and reduces the risk of injury.

Hydration :

Drink water before, during, and after your ruck. Carry water with you, especially for longer rucks. Staying hydrated is crucial for maintaining performance and preventing dehydration.

Listen to Your Body :

Pay attention to any discomfort or pain. Adjust the weight or distance as needed to avoid injury. If you experience persistent pain, take a break and consult a healthcare professional if necessary.

Intermediate and Advanced Training Plans

Once you have established a foundation with beginner rucking, you can progress to more structured and challenging training plans. These plans will help you build on your initial gains and take your rucking to the next level.

Intermediate Training Plan

Weeks 1-2

Frequency :

3 times per week. This allows for a balance between challenging your body and providing adequate recovery time.

Distance :

2-3 miles. This distance is manageable for intermediate ruckers and provides a solid workout.

Weight :

15-20% of body weight. This increment from beginner weights will continue to build strength and endurance.

Pace :

Maintain a steady, moderate pace. Focus on keeping a consistent speed throughout your ruck.

Terrain :

Start incorporating varied terrain, including hills and trails. This adds a new challenge and helps build different muscle groups.

Weeks 3-4

Frequency :

4 times per week. Increasing the frequency will further enhance your endurance and strength.

Distance :

3-4 miles. Gradually increasing the distance will push your limits and improve your stamina.

Weight :

20-25% of body weight. Continue to challenge yourself with incremental weight increases.

Pace :

Include intervals of faster walking or light jogging. Interval training can boost your cardiovascular fitness and calorie burn.

Terrain :

Use a mix of flat and hilly areas, increasing difficulty. This variation will keep your workouts interesting and challenging.

Weeks 5-6

Frequency :

4   times per week. Maintain this frequency to continue building endurance.

Distance :

4-5 miles. This distance will provide a robust workout without overextending your limits.

Weight :

25-30% of body weight. Pushing your weight limits will help build significant strength and resilience.

Pace :

Continue with interval training, adding more intensity. Try to incorporate short bursts of running if you feel comfortable.

Terrain :

Incorporate more rugged terrain with moderate inclines. This will test your balance and strengthen your stabilizing muscles.

Weeks 7-8

Frequency :

4-5 times per week. Adding an extra day will further increase your fitness levels.

Distance :

5-6 miles. By now, you should be comfortable with longer distances.

Weight :

30-35% of body weight. Continue to incrementally increase your weight as your strength builds.

Pace :

Maintain a brisk pace with regular intervals of jogging. This will keep your heart rate elevated and improve your cardiovascular endurance.

Terrain :

Challenge yourself with steeper inclines and more varied terrain. This will provide a comprehensive workout and prepare you for advanced rucking.

Advanced Training Plan

Weeks 1-2

Frequency :

4-5 times per week. This frequency will help you maintain a high level of fitness.

Distance :

6-7 miles. Pushing your distance will continue to build your endurance.

Weight :

35-40% of body weight. This weight level will challenge your strength and endurance.

Pace :

Include longer intervals of jogging or running. This will further improve your cardiovascular fitness.

Terrain :

Use challenging trails with varied elevation and rugged paths. This will test your skills and build resilience.

Weeks 3-4

Frequency :

5 times per week. Maintaining a high frequency will keep you at peak fitness.

Distance :

7-8 miles. Continue to push your distance for greater endurance gains.

Weight :

40-45% of body weight. This weight level will significantly challenge your strength and stamina.

Pace :

Increase the duration of jogging intervals. Longer intervals will improve your running endurance and overall fitness.

Terrain :

Focus on more difficult trails with steeper inclines and rocky paths. This will enhance your technical skills and build strength.

Weeks 5-6

Frequency :

5 times per week. Consistency is key for maintaining high fitness levels.

Distance :

8-9 miles. This distance will provide a challenging workout and improve your endurance.

Weight :

45-50% of body weight. Continue to push your weight limits for greater strength gains.

Pace :

Continue with advanced interval training, adding longer jogging segments. This will keep your workouts intense and effective.

Terrain :

Utilize highly challenging terrains to test your endurance and strength. This will prepare you for any rucking challenge.

Weeks 7-8

Frequency :

5-6 times per week. High frequency will ensure you maintain peak fitness levels.

Distance :

9-10 miles. By now, you should be comfortable with long distances and ready for extended rucks.

Weight :

50-55% of body weight. This weight level will significantly challenge your strength and endurance.

Pace :

Push your pace with longer periods of running. This will enhance your cardiovascular fitness and overall performance.

Terrain :

Focus on the most challenging trails, incorporating long inclines and technical paths. This will test your limits and build resilience.

Cross-Training: Complementary Exercises

To maximize the benefits of rucking and reduce the risk of injury, it's essential to incorporate crosstraining exercises into your routine. These exercises will help improve overall fitness, strength, flexibility, and recovery.

Strength Training Core

Planks :

Strengthen your core and improve stability. Hold for 30-60 seconds. Variations like side planks and plank leg lifts can add variety and challenge different muscles.

Russian Twists :

Improve rotational strength. Perform 15-20 reps per side. Use a medicine ball or weight to increase difficulty.

Leg Raises :

Enhance lower abdominal strength. Perform 15-20 reps. Keep your lower back pressed into the floor to avoid strain.

Legs

Squats :

Build leg strength and stability. Perform 3 sets of 1015 reps. Variations like goblet squats and single-leg squats can add challenge and improve balance.

Lunges :

Improve balance and leg strength. Perform 3 sets of 10-15 reps per leg. Try walking lunges or reverse lunges for variety.

Deadlifts :

Strengthen the posterior chain. Perform 3 sets of

8-12 reps. Use proper form to avoid injury, and consider variations like Romanian deadlifts.

Back and Shoulders

Pull-Ups :

Enhance upper body and back strength. Perform 3 sets of 5-10 reps. If you're a beginner, use resistance bands for assistance.

Rows :

Improve back and shoulder strength. Perform 3 sets of 10-15 reps. Variations like bent-over rows and single-arm rows can add variety.

Shoulder Presses :

Build shoulder strength. Perform 3 sets of 10-12 reps. Try seated or standing variations for different challenges.

Cardiovascular Exercises

Running

Short Runs :

Improve cardiovascular fitness and leg strength. Start with 1-2 miles, gradually increasing. Use different paces to build endurance and speed.

Interval Training :

Alternate between sprinting and walking/jogging to enhance stamina. For example, sprint for 30 seconds, then walk for 1 minute. Repeat for 20-30 minutes.

Cycling

Outdoor Cycling :

Provides a low-impact cardiovascular workout and strengthens leg muscles. Aim for 30-60 minutes. Include hills to build strength and endurance.

Stationary Cycling :

Use interval training to increase intensity and improve endurance. For example, alternate between high resistance for 1 minute and low resistance for 2 minutes.

Swimming

Laps :

Offers a full-body workout with minimal joint impact. Swim for 20-30 minutes. Vary your strokes to work different muscle groups.

Drills :

Focus on different strokes to improve overall swimming ability and fitness. For example, practice freestyle, backstroke, and breaststroke.

Flexibility and Mobility

Yoga

Flexibility :

Enhances flexibility, balance, and mental focus. Practice for 20-30 minutes. Focus on poses that stretch the muscles used in rucking, like hamstrings and hip flexors.

Recovery :

Helps in muscle recovery and reduces soreness. Incorporate restorative poses and deep breathing exercises.

Dynamic Stretching

Pre-Ruck :

Prepares muscles for activity and improves range of motion. Spend 5-10 minutes on dynamic stretches like leg swings and arm circles.

Foam Rolling

Post-Ruck :

Relieves muscle tension and aids in recovery. Spend 10-15 minutes on foam rolling. Focus on areas like the calves, quads, and back.

Balance and Stability

Balance Drills

Single-Leg Stands :

Improve balance and stability. Hold for 30-60 seconds per leg. Close your eyes or stand on a soft surface to increase difficulty.

Balance Board Exercises :

Enhance balance and core strength. Perform exercises like squats and tilts on a balance board.

By incorporating these cross-training exercises into your routine, you will enhance your rucking performance, reduce the risk of injury, and achieve a well-rounded fitness level. Whether you are a beginner, intermediate, or advanced rucker, crosstraining will help you reach your goals and enjoy the many benefits of this versatile and effective workout.

First Steps to Rucking: A Beginner's Guide

1. Understanding Rucking :

   - Definition : Rucking involves carrying a weighted backpack while walking or hiking. It's a simple yet effective workout that builds muscle, improves endurance, and boosts cardiovascular health.

   - Benefits : Strengthens legs, core, and back muscles, improves posture, burns calories, and can be done virtually anywhere with minimal equipment.

2. Getting Started :

   - Choosing Your Gear :

   - Backpack : Select a durable, comfortable backpack with padded straps and a waist belt. It should fit snugly to avoid shifting while you walk.

- Weight : Start with a weight that is 10-15% of your body weight. You can use weight plates, sandbags, or even household items like water bottles.

- Footwear : Invest in supportive, comfortable shoes designed for walking or hiking. Ensure they have good arch support and cushioning.

- Basic Technique :

- Posture : Stand tall with your shoulders back, core engaged, and head up. Avoid leaning forward or backward excessively.

- Walking Form : Walk with a natural stride, keeping your steps steady and smooth. Use your arms for balance and rhythm.

- Starting Routine :

- Duration : Begin with short rucks of 20-30 minutes.

- Frequency : Aim for 2-3 times per week.

- Progression : Gradually increase the weight and duration as your fitness improves.

3. Safety Tips :

   - Warm-Up and Cool-Down : Perform a light warm-up before starting and cool down with stretching afterward.

   - Hydration : Drink water before, during, and after your ruck.

   - Listen to Your Body : Pay attention to any discomfort or pain. Adjust weight or distance as needed to avoid injury.

Intermediate and Advanced Training Plans

As you become more comfortable with rucking, you can increase the intensity and complexity of your workouts. Here are structured training plans for intermediate and advanced levels:

Intermediate Training Plan :

1. Weeks 1-2 :

   - Frequency : 3 times per week.

   - Distance : 2-3 miles.

   - Weight : 15-20% of body weight.

- Pace : Moderate, maintaining a steady and brisk walk.

- Terrain : Mix of flat and slightly hilly areas.

2. Weeks 3-4 :

  - Frequency : 4 times per week.

  - Distance : 3-4 miles.

  - Weight : 20-25% of body weight.

  - Pace : Include intervals of faster walking or light jogging.

  - Terrain : Incorporate more varied terrain with moderate inclines.

3. Weeks 5-6 :

  - Frequency : 4 times per week.

  - Distance : 4-5 miles.

  - Weight : 25-30% of body weight.

  - Pace : Continue with interval training, including steeper inclines.

  - Terrain : Challenge yourself with more rugged terrain and longer inclines.

Advanced Training Plan :

1. Weeks 1-2 :

  - Frequency : 4-5 times per week.

  - Distance : 5-6 miles.

  - Weight : 30-35% of body weight.

  - Pace : Maintain a brisk pace with regular intervals of jogging.

  - Terrain : Include challenging trails with varied elevation.

2. Weeks 3-4 :

  - Frequency : 5 times per week.

  - Distance : 6-8 miles.

  - Weight : 35-40% of body weight.

  - Pace : Incorporate longer intervals of jogging or running.

  - Terrain : Explore more difficult trails with steep and rocky paths.

3. Weeks 5-6 :

- Frequency : 5 times per week.

- Distance : 8-10 miles.

- Weight : 40-45% of body weight.

- Pace : Continue with advanced interval training, including sustained jogging segments.

- Terrain : Focus on highly challenging terrains to test your endurance and strength.

Cross-Training: Complementary Exercises

Incorporating cross-training exercises into your routine can enhance your overall fitness and prevent overuse injuries. Here are some complementary exercises for ruckers:

1. Strength Training :

   - Core : Planks, Russian twists, leg raises.

   - Legs : Squats, lunges, deadlifts.

   - Back and Shoulders : Pull-ups, rows, shoulder presses.

2. Cardiovascular Exercises :

   - Running : Improves cardiovascular fitness and leg strength.

   - Cycling : Provides a low-impact cardiovascular workout and strengthens leg muscles.

   - Swimming : Offers a full-body workout and is excellent for active recovery.

3. Flexibility and Mobility :

   - Yoga : Enhances flexibility, balance, and mental focus.

   - Dynamic Stretching : Prepares muscles for activity and improves range of motion.

   - Foam Rolling : Relieves muscle tension and aids in recovery.

4. Balance and Stability :

   - Balance Drills : Single-leg stands, balance board exercises.

   - Stability Ball Workouts : Incorporate exercises like stability ball push-ups and hamstring curls to improve core stability.

CHAPTER 6

Nutrition and Hydration for Ruckers

Nutrition and hydration are fundamental aspects of any physical activity, and rucking is no exception. Whether you're a novice or an experienced rucker, understanding what to eat and drink before, during, and after your workouts can significantly impact your performance and recovery. This guide will delve into the essentials of nutrition and hydration for ruckers, providing comprehensive information on macronutrients, hydration strategies, meal planning, supplements, and more.

The Importance of Nutrition for Ruckers

Proper nutrition fuels your body, aids in muscle repair, and enhances overall performance. For ruckers, a balanced diet ensures sustained energy levels, reduces the risk of injury, and promotes quicker recovery. Let's break down the key components of a rucker's diet:

Macronutrients

Carbohydrates

Carbohydrates are the primary energy source for ruckers. They are stored as glycogen in the muscles and liver, which your body uses during prolonged physical activity.

-       Complex Carbohydrates   : Include whole grains, brown rice, quinoa, oats, and sweet potatoes in your diet. These provide sustained energy and keep you feeling full longer.

-       Simple Carbohydrates   : Consume fruits, vegetables, and dairy products for quick energy. These are also essential for replenishing glycogen stores post-ruck.

Proteins

Proteins are crucial for muscle repair and growth. They help rebuild muscle fibers that are broken down during rucking.

-        Lean Proteins : Incorporate chicken, turkey, lean beef, and fish into your meals. These provide essential amino acids for muscle repair.

-        Plant-Based Proteins : Include beans, lentils, tofu, and tempeh if you follow a vegetarian or vegan diet.

Fats

Fats are a vital energy source, especially for longduration activities. They also aid in the absorption of fat-soluble vitamins (A, D, E, and K).

-        Healthy Fats : Focus on avocados, nuts, seeds, olive oil, and fatty fish like salmon. These fats support overall health and provide sustained energy.

Micronutrients

Vitamins and Minerals

Ruckers need a variety of vitamins and minerals to support metabolic functions, bone health, and immune function.

-       Calcium : Essential for bone health. Found in dairy products, leafy greens, and fortified plant milks.

-       Iron : Important for oxygen transport in the blood. Sources include red meat, poultry, beans, and fortified cereals.

-       Magnesium : Supports muscle function and recovery. Found in nuts, seeds, whole grains, and leafy greens.

-       Vitamin D : Aids in calcium absorption and bone health. Obtain from sun exposure, fatty fish, and fortified foods.

-       Vitamin C : Supports immune function and collagen production. Found in citrus fruits, berries, and bell peppers.

Hydration Strategies for Ruckers

Proper hydration is critical for maintaining performance and preventing dehydration during rucking. Here's how to manage your fluid intake effectively:

Pre-Ruck Hydration

-       Start Hydrated : Drink 16-20 ounces of water 2-3 hours before your ruck. This ensures your body is well-hydrated at the start.

-       Electrolytes   : Consider a beverage with electrolytes if you'll be rucking for an extended period. Electrolytes help maintain fluid balance and prevent cramps.

During-Ruck Hydration

-       Regular Sips : Drink 7-10 ounces of water every 20 minutes. Adjust this amount based on the intensity and duration of your ruck, as well as the weather conditions.

-       Electrolyte Replenishment : For rucks lasting more than an hour, consume a drink with electrolytes to replace lost sodium, potassium, and other essential minerals.

Post-Ruck Hydration

-

Rehydration : Drink 16-24 ounces of water for every pound lost during your ruck. Weighing yourself before and after can help determine how much fluid you've lost.

-        Recovery Drinks : Consider a recovery drink that includes both carbohydrates and electrolytes to replenish glycogen stores and aid in muscle recovery.

Meal Planning for Ruckers

A well-structured meal plan ensures you get the right balance of nutrients to support your rucking activities. Here's a sample meal plan to guide you:

Pre-Ruck Meal

Timing : 2-3 hours before your ruck

Example :

- Grilled chicken breast

-

-

Quinoa or brown rice

Steamed vegetables (broccoli, carrots, and bell peppers)

- A small serving of fruit (banana or apple)

During-Ruck Snacks

Timing : Every 45-60 minutes during your ruck

Example :

- Energy gels or chews

- A handful of nuts and dried fruit

- A banana or apple slices

Post-Ruck Meal

Timing : Within 30 minutes to 2 hours after your ruck

-

-

Example :

Lean protein (grilled salmon or chicken)

Sweet potato or whole grain pasta

- Leafy green salad with olive oil and lemon dressing

- Greek yogurt with honey and berries

Daily Meal Plan

Breakfast :

- Oatmeal with berries, nuts, and a drizzle of honey

- Scrambled eggs with spinach and tomatoes

- A glass of low-fat milk or a dairy-free alternative

Lunch :

- Turkey and avocado wrap on whole grain tortilla

- Side of mixed greens with a light vinaigrette

- A piece of fruit (orange or pear)

-

-

Dinner :

- Grilled tofu or tempeh

- Brown rice or quinoa

-

Steamed vegetables (asparagus, Brussels sprouts, and zucchini)

Snacks :

- Greek yogurt with a handful of granola

- Hummus with carrot and celery sticks

- A smoothie made with spinach, banana, almond milk, and protein powder

Supplements for Ruckers

While a balanced diet should provide most of the nutrients you need, supplements can help fill any gaps and support your performance and recovery.

Protein Supplements

Whey Protein : Quickly absorbed and ideal for post-ruck recovery. It provides all essential amino acids for muscle repair.

Plant-Based Protein : Suitable for those who prefer a vegetarian or vegan option. Look for blends that include pea, rice, and hemp proteins.

Electrolyte Supplements

Electrolyte Tablets : Convenient and easy to carry. Drop them into your water bottle to maintain electrolyte balance during long rucks.

Electrolyte Powders : Mix with water for a quick electrolyte boost. Look for options with low sugar content.

Vitamins and Minerals

Multivitamins : Ensure you get a broad range of essential vitamins and minerals. Choose a highquality multivitamin tailored to your needs.

Vitamin D : Especially important if you have limited sun exposure. Supports bone health and immune function.

Magnesium : Aids in muscle recovery and helps prevent cramps. Available in tablet or powder form.

Special Considerations for Rucking Nutrition

Weight Management

Rucking can be an effective way to manage your weight, but it's essential to balance your caloric intake with your activity level.

-        Caloric Intake   : Ensure you're consuming enough calories to fuel your rucks without overeating. Use a calorie-tracking app to monitor your intake.

-        Macronutrient Balance : Aim for a balanced diet with appropriate ratios of carbohydrates, proteins, and fats. Adjust these ratios based on your goals (e.g., higher protein for muscle building).

Dealing with Heat and Cold

Hot Weather :

-       Hydration : Increase your fluid intake to compensate for sweat loss. Consider adding more electrolytes to prevent dehydration.

-       Cooling Foods : Consume foods with high water content, such as watermelon, cucumbers, and oranges. These help keep you hydrated and cool.

-       Timing : Ruck during cooler parts of the day, such as early morning or late evening, to avoid extreme heat.

Cold Weather :

-       Warm Foods : Incorporate warm meals like soups and stews. These provide comfort and essential nutrients.

-       Hydration : Don't neglect hydration, even if you don't feel as thirsty. Cold weather can still lead to dehydration.

-       Energy-Dense Foods : Increase your intake of healthy fats, such as nuts and avocados, to provide sustained energy in the cold.

Practical Tips for Rucking Nutrition

Meal Prep

-        Batch Cooking : Prepare meals in advance to save time and ensure you have nutritious options ready. Cook large portions of grains, proteins, and vegetables that can be easily reheated.

-        Portable Snacks : Keep healthy snacks on hand, such as nuts, seeds, and dried fruit, for quick energy boosts during your rucks.

Experimentation

-        Test Foods and Drinks : Experiment with different foods and drinks during training to see what works best for you. Pay attention to how your body reacts and make adjustments as needed.

-        Race-Day Nutrition : If you participate in events, practice your race-day nutrition strategy during training to avoid surprises.

Listening to Your Body

-        Hunger and Fullness : Pay attention to your body's hunger and fullness cues. Eat when you're hungry and stop when you're satisfied.

-       Recovery Needs : Adjust your nutrition based on your recovery needs. After particularly strenuous rucks, focus on higher protein intake and adequate hydration.

Fueling Your Body: Essential Nutrition Tips

Proper nutrition is the cornerstone of any successful fitness regimen, and rucking is no exception. To perform at your best and recover effectively, it's crucial to fuel your body with the right nutrients. This guide will provide you with essential nutrition tips, the importance of staying hydrated, and effective strategies for using supplements and promoting recovery.

Essential Nutrition Tips for Ruckers

Understanding the basics of nutrition can help you make informed choices about what to eat before, during, and after your rucking sessions. Here are some key principles:

1. Balance Your Macronutrients

Your diet should include a healthy balance of carbohydrates, proteins, and fats:

-	Carbohydrates : These are your primary source of energy, especially for endurance activities like rucking. Opt for complex carbs such as whole grains, legumes, and vegetables, which provide sustained energy and stabilize blood sugar levels.

-	Proteins : Essential for muscle repair and growth. Incorporate lean proteins like chicken, turkey, fish, eggs, and plant-based sources such as beans, lentils, and tofu.

-	Fats : Healthy fats are vital for energy and nutrient absorption. Include sources like avocados, nuts, seeds, and olive oil.

2. Prioritize Micronutrients

Vitamins and minerals are crucial for overall health and performance. Ensure you get a variety of micronutrients by consuming a wide range of fruits, vegetables, nuts, and seeds. Key micronutrients for ruckers include:

-        Calcium : Supports bone health. Found in dairy products, leafy greens, and fortified plant milks.

-        Iron : Essential for oxygen transport in the blood. Sources include red meat, poultry, beans, and fortified cereals.

-        Magnesium : Supports muscle function and recovery. Found in nuts, seeds, whole grains, and leafy greens.

-        Vitamin D : Aids in calcium absorption and bone health. Obtain from sun exposure, fatty fish, and fortified foods.

3. Plan Your Meals Around Your Rucking Schedule

Timing your meals correctly can enhance performance and recovery:

-        Pre-Ruck Meal : Eat a balanced meal 2-3 hours before your ruck to fuel your body with carbohydrates and proteins. A good example is a chicken and quinoa bowl with steamed vegetables.

-        During-Ruck Snacks : For longer rucks, bring easy-to-digest snacks like energy gels, bananas, or a mix of nuts and dried fruit.

-        Post-Ruck Meal : Consume a meal rich in proteins and carbohydrates within 30 minutes to 2 hours after your ruck to replenish glycogen stores and aid muscle recovery. A grilled salmon with sweet potato and a side salad is an excellent option.

4. Listen to Your Body

Pay attention to your hunger and energy levels. Eat when you're hungry, and avoid overeating. Adjust your intake based on the intensity and duration of your rucking sessions.

Staying Hydrated: The Importance of Water

Hydration is crucial for maintaining performance and preventing dehydration. Here's how to manage your fluid intake effectively:

1. Pre-Ruck Hydration

-       Start Hydrated : Drink 16-20 ounces of water 2-3 hours before your ruck. This ensures your body is well-hydrated at the start.

-       Electrolytes   : Consider a beverage with electrolytes if you'll be rucking for an extended period. Electrolytes help maintain fluid balance and prevent cramps.

2. During-Ruck Hydration

-       Regular Sips : Drink 7-10 ounces of water every 20 minutes. Adjust this amount based on the intensity and duration of your ruck, as well as the weather conditions.

-       Electrolyte Replenishment : For rucks lasting more than an hour, consume a drink with electrolytes to replace lost sodium, potassium, and other essential minerals.

3. Post-Ruck Hydration

-       Rehydration : Drink 16-24 ounces of water for every pound lost during your ruck. Weighing yourself before and after can help determine how much fluid you've lost.

-       Recovery Drinks : Consider a recovery drink that includes both carbohydrates and electrolytes to replenish glycogen stores and aid in muscle recovery.

4. Tips for Staying Hydrated

-        Carry a Water Bottle : Always have a water bottle with you, and sip water throughout the day.

-        Monitor Urine Color   : Pale yellow urine typically indicates proper hydration, while dark yellow may signal dehydration.

-        Hydrate with Foods : Consume foods with high water content, such as cucumbers, watermelon, and oranges, to help meet your hydration needs.

Supplements and Recovery Strategies

Supplements can help fill any nutritional gaps and support your performance and recovery. Here are some commonly used supplements and effective recovery strategies:

1. Protein Supplements

-        Whey Protein : Quickly absorbed and ideal for post-ruck recovery. It provides all essential amino acids for muscle repair.

-       Plant-Based Protein : Suitable for those who prefer a vegetarian or vegan option. Look for blends that include pea, rice, and hemp proteins.

2. Electrolyte Supplements

-       Electrolyte Tablets : Convenient and easy to carry. Drop them into your water bottle to maintain electrolyte balance during long rucks.

-       Electrolyte Powders : Mix with water for a quick electrolyte boost. Look for options with low sugar content.

3. Vitamins and Minerals

-       Multivitamins : Ensure you get a broad range of essential vitamins and minerals. Choose a highquality multivitamin tailored to your needs.

-       Vitamin D : Especially important if you have limited sun exposure. Supports bone health and immune function.

-       Magnesium : Aids in muscle recovery and helps prevent cramps. Available in tablet or powder form.

4. Recovery Strategies

-        Rest and Sleep : Prioritize 7-9 hours of sleep per night to allow your body to repair and rebuild muscle tissue. Rest days are also essential to prevent overtraining and reduce the risk of injury.

-        Foam Rolling and Stretching : Incorporate foam rolling and stretching into your routine to alleviate muscle tension, improve flexibility, and reduce soreness.

-        Active Recovery : Engage in low-intensity activities like walking, swimming, or yoga on rest days to promote blood flow and aid in recovery.

-        Massage Therapy : Regular massages can help alleviate muscle soreness, reduce tension, and improve circulation.

5. Meal Timing for Recovery

- Post-Ruck Nutrition : Consume a meal or snack rich in carbohydrates and proteins within 30 minutes to 2 hours after your ruck. This helps replenish glycogen stores and supports muscle repair.

- Evening Snack : Have a light snack before bed that includes protein and healthy fats, such as

Greek yogurt with nuts or a small smoothie. This provides your body with the nutrients it needs for overnight recovery.

Putting It All Together: A Sample Day of Nutrition and Hydration for Ruckers

Here's a sample day to illustrate how you can integrate these tips into your routine:

Morning (Pre-Ruck)

- Breakfast   : Oatmeal with berries, nuts, and a drizzle of honey. A glass of low-fat milk or a dairyfree alternative.

- Hydration   : 16-20 ounces of water 2-3 hours before rucking. Consider a drink with electrolytes if rucking for an extended period.

Mid-Morning (During Ruck)

- Snack : A banana or an energy gel.

- Hydration   : 7-10 ounces of water every 20 minutes. Add electrolyte tablets if needed.

Afternoon (Post-Ruck)

- Lunch : Grilled chicken breast with quinoa and steamed vegetables. A small serving of fruit.
- Hydration : 16-24 ounces of water for every pound lost during rucking. Consider a recovery drink with carbohydrates and electrolytes.

Evening

- Dinner : Grilled salmon with sweet potato and a side salad with olive oil and lemon dressing.
- Snack : Greek yogurt with a handful of granola and a small piece of dark chocolate.

Throughout the Day

- Hydration : Sip water regularly and monitor urine color. Incorporate hydrating foods like cucumbers and oranges into your meals.

By following these essential nutrition tips, maintaining proper hydration, and utilizing effective supplements and recovery strategies, you can enhance your rucking performance and overall wellbeing. Remember, consistency is key, and listening to your body's needs will help you achieve your fitness goals while enjoying the benefits of this challenging and rewarding activity.

CHAPTER 7

Preparing for Rucking Events and Competitions

Preparing for Rucking Events and Competitions

Participating in rucking events and competitions requires careful preparation to ensure peak performance and safety. Whether you're a novice rucker or an experienced participant, following a structured plan can help you achieve your goals and enjoy the event. This guide will provide comprehensive tips on training, nutrition, gear selection, mental preparation, and recovery strategies to help you get ready for your next rucking event or competition.

Training for Rucking Events

1. Build a Solid Foundation

Before diving into intense training, ensure you have a strong base of fitness. Focus on general cardiovascular conditioning and strength training.

-       Cardio Workouts : Incorporate activities like running, cycling, or swimming to build cardiovascular endurance.

-       Strength Training   : Target major muscle groups with exercises like squats, lunges, deadlifts, and push-ups to enhance overall strength and stability.

2. Gradual Progression

Increase the intensity and duration of your rucking sessions gradually to avoid injury and build stamina.

-       Increase Weight Slowly : Start with a light load and gradually increase the weight in your rucksack. Aim for 10-20% of your body weight initially and incrementally add more weight.

-       Extend Distance and Duration   : Gradually extend the distance and duration of your rucking sessions.

Aim to increase your distance by no more than 10% per week.

3. Specific Training for the Event

Tailor your training to match the specific demands of the event.

-        Simulate Event Conditions : Train on similar terrain and under similar weather conditions as the event. If the event involves hills or trails, incorporate those into your training.

-        Practice with Full Gear : Train with the same gear you'll use during the event, including your rucksack, boots, and clothing. This helps you get accustomed to the weight and feel of the gear.

4. Incorporate Interval Training

Interval training can enhance your cardiovascular fitness and help you handle varying intensities during the event.

High-Intensity Intervals : Include sessions where you alternate between high-intensity efforts and lowintensity recovery periods. For example, alternate between fast-paced rucking and a slower pace.

-   Hill Intervals : If the event involves elevation changes, practice hill intervals by rucking up and down hills to build leg strength and endurance.

5. Cross-Training

Incorporate complementary exercises to improve overall fitness and reduce the risk of overuse injuries.

-       Swimming : Provides a low-impact cardiovascular workout and helps improve lung capacity.

-       Cycling : Builds leg strength and endurance without the impact of rucking.

-       Yoga and Stretching : Enhances flexibility, reduces muscle tension, and improves balance.

Nutrition and Hydration

-

Proper nutrition and hydration are crucial for optimal performance during rucking events.

1. Pre-Event Nutrition

Fuel your body with the right nutrients in the days leading up to the event.

-       Carbohydrate Loading   : Increase your carbohydrate intake 2-3 days before the event to maximize glycogen stores. Focus on complex carbohydrates like whole grains, pasta, and vegetables.

-       Balanced Meals   : Ensure your meals are wellbalanced, including lean proteins, healthy fats, and plenty of fruits and vegetables.

2. Hydration

Maintain proper hydration before, during, and after the event.

Pre-Event Hydration : Start hydrating well before the event. Drink plenty of water in the days leading up to the competition.

-        During the Event : Drink water regularly, and consider electrolyte drinks to replace lost minerals. Aim to drink 7-10 ounces of water every 20 minutes.

-        Post-Event   Hydration   :   Rehydrate immediately after the event. Drink 16-24 ounces of water for every pound lost during the event.

3. Nutrition During the Event

Fuel your body during the event to maintain energy levels.

-        Easy-to-Digest Foods   : Consume energy gels, bars, or fruits like bananas and oranges that are easy to digest and provide quick energy.

-        Small, Frequent Snacks : Eat small amounts at regular intervals to keep your energy levels steady.

4. Post-Event Nutrition

-

Focus on recovery with a balanced meal after the event.

-       Protein and Carbohydrates   : Consume a meal rich in proteins and carbohydrates to replenish glycogen stores and aid muscle recovery. Consider options like a chicken and vegetable stir-fry with brown rice.

-       Recovery Drinks : Consider a recovery drink that includes both carbohydrates and proteins to kickstart the recovery process.

Selecting the Right Gear

Choosing the right gear is essential for comfort and performance during rucking events.

1. Rucksack

Select a rucksack that fits well and can comfortably carry your gear.

Fit and Comfort : Ensure the rucksack has adjustable straps and a padded back panel for comfort. The weight should be evenly distributed.

-     Capacity : Choose a rucksack with enough capacity to hold your gear, but avoid overloading it. Aim for a balance between carrying essentials and maintaining a manageable weight.

2. Footwear

Proper footwear is crucial for preventing blisters and ensuring comfort.

-     Rucking Boots : Invest in a good pair of rucking boots that provide support and durability. Look for boots with a sturdy sole, ankle support, and breathable materials.

-     Socks : Wear moisture-wicking socks to prevent blisters. Consider double-layer socks or liner socks for added protection.

3. Clothing

-

Dress appropriately for the weather and terrain.

- Moisture-Wicking Fabrics : Wear moisturewicking and breathable clothing to keep you dry and comfortable.

- Layering : Dress in layers to adjust to changing weather conditions. Consider a base layer, an insulating layer, and a waterproof outer layer.

- Sun Protection : Wear a hat and apply sunscreen to protect yourself from the sun.

4. Additional Gear

Pack essential gear for safety and comfort.

- Hydration System : Use a hydration bladder or carry water bottles to ensure you stay hydrated.

- Navigation Tools : Carry a map, compass, or GPS device to stay on course.

- First Aid Kit : Include basic first aid supplies such as bandages, antiseptic wipes, and blister treatments.

Emergency Gear : Carry a whistle, multi-tool, and a small emergency blanket.

Mental Preparation

Mental preparation is just as important as physical training for rucking events.

1. Set Realistic Goals

Set achievable goals for the event based on your training and fitness level.

-      Performance Goals   : Define specific performance goals, such as completing the event within a certain time or maintaining a steady pace.

-      Process Goals : Focus on process-oriented goals, like maintaining proper form, staying hydrated, and pacing yourself.

2. Visualization

-

Use visualization techniques to mentally prepare for the event.

-       Visualize Success : Picture yourself successfully completing the event. Visualize the route, the challenges, and how you'll overcome them.

-       Positive Self-Talk : Use positive affirmations and self-talk to build confidence and stay motivated.

3. Stay Focused and Positive

Maintain a positive mindset and stay focused during the event.

-       Break It Down : Break the event into smaller, manageable sections. Focus on one section at a time rather than the entire event.

-       Stay Motivated   : Use motivational techniques, such as listening to music, thinking about why you're participating, and recalling past successes.

Recovery Strategies

Proper recovery is essential for preventing injury and promoting long-term performance.

1. Cool Down

Cool down immediately after the event to aid recovery.

-       Light Activity : Engage in light activity such as walking or stretching to gradually lower your heart rate.

-       Foam Rolling : Use a foam roller to massage sore muscles and improve blood flow.

2. Post-Event Nutrition

Consume a balanced meal within two hours after the event to support recovery.

- Protein and Carbohydrates : Include lean proteins and complex carbohydrates in your post-event meal to replenish glycogen stores and promote muscle repair.

-

Hydration : Continue to hydrate after the event to replace lost fluids and electrolytes.

3. Rest and Sleep

Prioritize rest and sleep in the days following the event.

-       Active Recovery : Engage in low-intensity activities like walking, yoga, or swimming to promote blood flow and aid recovery.

-       Quality Sleep : Aim for 7-9 hours of quality sleep per night to allow your body to repair and rebuild.

4. Monitor Your Body

Pay attention to how your body feels and address any issues promptly.

-

- Injury Prevention : If you experience pain or discomfort, take time to rest and recover. Consult a healthcare professional if necessary.

Ongoing Care : Incorporate regular stretching, foam rolling, and massage into your routine to prevent muscle tightness and promote flexibility.

Overview of Popular Rucking Challenges

Rucking challenges are designed to test endurance, strength, and mental fortitude. They vary widely in terms of difficulty, terrain, and goals. Understanding these challenges can help you prepare effectively and choose events that match your interests and abilities. Here's an overview of some popular rucking challenges:

1. GORUCK Challenges

Overview : GORUCK is one of the most wellknown rucking organizations, offering a variety of events. Their challenges include rucks of varying distances and durations, often with a militaryinspired twist.

-

Popular Events :

   GORUCK Light : A 4-5 hour event covering 6-10 miles. It includes team-building exercises and challenges.

-       GORUCK Tough   : A 10-12 hour event covering 15-20 miles. Participants face physical and mental challenges, including carrying heavy weights and completing team tasks.

-       GORUCK Heavy : A 24-hour event covering 3040 miles. This is the most grueling of the GORUCK events, combining endurance with team-based problem-solving.

Challenges :

-       Teamwork and Leadership : Many GORUCK events emphasize teamwork, leadership, and problem-solving under pressure.

-       Varied Terrain : Challenges often take place in urban, rural, or mountainous environments, requiring adaptability.

   2. The Hike for Heroes

-

Overview : This is a charitable rucking event that typically involves hiking long distances to raise funds for military and first responder charities.

Popular Events :

-       Hike for Heroes 50K : A 50-kilometer hike that tests endurance and fundraising abilities. Participants often hike with a weighted rucksack to increase the challenge.

-       Local Hike for Heroes Events : Smaller, community-based hikes that support local charities.

Challenges :

-       Fundraising   : Participants are usually required to raise a certain amount of money for charity, adding a fundraising component to the physical challenge.

-       Endurance : These events often require long hours of hiking, sometimes over challenging terrain.

3.   The GoRuck Star Course

Overview : The GoRuck Star Course is an annual event that challenges participants to complete a 50mile ruck in 20 hours.

Popular Event :

-        GoRuck Star Course 50-Miler : Participants carry a 30-pound rucksack and navigate checkpoints while dealing with physical and mental challenges.

Challenges :

-        Navigation : Participants must navigate using maps and compass, adding a navigational element to the physical challenge.

-        Endurance and Speed : Completing 50 miles in 20 hours requires a high level of endurance and speed.

4.   The Ultimate Ruck Challenge

Overview : This challenge often involves rucking a set number of miles within a specific timeframe, with the option to scale up based on participant ability.

Popular Event :

-        24-Hour Ultimate Ruck : Participants ruck as many miles as possible within 24 hours, typically with a weighted pack.

Challenges :

-        Mental Toughness   : Rucking for extended periods tests mental resilience and pain tolerance.

-        Self-Paced : Participants must manage their own pace and rest breaks to optimize performance.

Training for Success: Event Preparation Tips

Proper preparation is crucial for success in rucking events. Here are some training and preparation tips to help you excel:

1.   Develop a Structured Training Plan

Build Endurance :

-        Progressive Long Rucks : Gradually increase the distance and weight of your rucks. Start with shorter distances and lighter weights, and slowly build up.

-        Back-to-Back Rucks : Practice doing rucks on consecutive days to simulate event conditions and build endurance.

Increase Strength :

-        Strength Training : Focus on exercises that build leg strength, core stability, and overall endurance. Squats, lunges, deadlifts, and step-ups are particularly beneficial.

-        Weight Training : Incorporate weight training to strengthen muscles used in rucking. Include exercises that target the shoulders, back, and hips.

Improve Cardiovascular Fitness :

-        Cross-Training : Engage in activities like running, cycling, or swimming to improve cardiovascular fitness and stamina.

-        Interval Training : Include high-intensity interval training (HIIT) to boost your cardiovascular capacity and simulate the varying intensities of a rucking event.

2. Simulate Event Conditions

Terrain Training :

-        Train on Similar Terrain   : If your event involves hills or trails, train on similar terrain to acclimate your body to the conditions.

-

Weight Simulation : Train with the same weight and gear you'll use during the event to get accustomed to the load.

Practice Navigation :

-        Map Reading : Practice reading maps and using a compass if the event involves navigation.

-        Route Familiarization : Familiarize yourself with the event route, if possible, to reduce uncertainty on race day.

3.   Optimize Nutrition and Hydration

Pre-Event Nutrition :

-        Carbohydrate Loading   :   Increase carbohydrate intake in the days leading up to the event to maximize glycogen stores.

-        Balanced Meals : Ensure your meals are wellbalanced, including proteins, fats, and carbohydrates.

During the Event :

-

Hydration : Stay hydrated by drinking water regularly and consuming electrolyte drinks if necessary.

- Energy Snacks : Pack easy-to-digest snacks that provide quick energy, such as energy gels, bars, or fruits.

Post-Event Recovery :

- Recovery Meal : Consume a meal rich in proteins and carbohydrates within two hours after the event to aid recovery.

- Hydration : Rehydrate to replace lost fluids and electrolytes.

4. Prepare Mentally

Set Goals :

- Performance Goals : Set realistic goals based on your training and fitness level.

- Process Goals : Focus on process-oriented goals, such as maintaining proper form and pacing.

-

Visualization and Mental Rehearsal :

Visualize Success : Picture yourself successfully completing the event to build confidence and reduce anxiety.

-        Positive Self-Talk   : Use affirmations and positive self-talk to stay motivated and focused.

Stories from the Field: Rucking Experiences

Hearing from individuals who have participated in rucking events can provide valuable insights and inspiration. Here are some stories from the field:

1. Overcoming the Odds

Participant : Sarah, an amateur rucker

Story : Sarah was new to rucking and decided to participate in a local 50K rucking event to challenge herself. Despite struggling with the weight and

273

-

distance initially, she focused on her training, gradually increasing her endurance and strength. On the day of the event, Sarah maintained a steady pace and used mental strategies to stay positive. She finished the event, feeling a great sense of accomplishment and newfound confidence in her abilities.

Key Takeaway   : Sarah's story highlights the importance of gradual training, mental resilience, and the rewards of pushing through challenges.

2. Teamwork and Camaraderie

Participant : Mike, a veteran rucker

Story : Mike participated in a GORUCK Tough event, which involved carrying heavy weights and completing team-based challenges. The event emphasized teamwork and leadership, and Mike found that the camaraderie and support from fellow participants were crucial to overcoming the physical and mental demands. The shared experience and teamwork not only helped him complete the event but also forged lasting friendships.

Key Takeaway : Mike's story underscores the value of teamwork and community in rucking events, demonstrating how collaboration can enhance the experience and success.

3. Charity and Purpose

Participant : Laura, a rucker for charity

Story : Laura took part in a Hike for Heroes event to support military and first responder charities. The challenge involved hiking long distances with a weighted pack, and Laura's motivation was fueled by the cause she was supporting. Despite the physical strain, the sense of purpose and the impact of her fundraising efforts kept her going. Laura completed the hike and felt proud of both her personal achievement and the difference she made through her efforts.

Key Takeaway : Laura's story highlights the motivational power of participating in charity events, where the cause can provide extra drive and fulfillment.

CHAPTER 8
Rucking for Everyone

Rucking for Weight Loss

Rucking is a powerful tool for weight loss, offering a unique combination of cardiovascular and strength training that burns calories efficiently. Here's how rucking can be an effective part of a weight loss journey:

Caloric Burn and Metabolism Boost

Carrying weight while walking increases the intensity of the exercise, leading to higher caloric expenditure. For example, a 30-minute walk at a moderate pace might burn around 150 calories for an average person, but adding a 20-pound rucksack can increase that burn significantly. This additional calorie consumption helps create a caloric deficit, essential for weight loss.

Rucking also engages major muscle groups, including the legs, core, and back. This engagement promotes muscle growth and maintenance, which in turn can boost metabolism. A higher resting metabolic rate means your body burns more calories even at rest, supporting long-term weight management.

Building Sustainable Habits

Rucking is a sustainable and enjoyable form of exercise that can easily be integrated into daily routines. Unlike high-intensity workouts that may be intimidating or unsustainable for some, rucking offers a low-impact alternative that can be done almost anywhere, from urban environments to nature trails.

Consistency is key in any weight loss plan. Setting a routine, whether it's a daily morning ruck or a weekly group ruck, can help solidify the habit. Start with achievable goals, such as rucking for 30 minutes a few times a week, and gradually increase the duration, weight, or frequency as your fitness level improves.

Mindful Nutrition and Hydration

While rucking alone can aid in weight loss, combining it with mindful nutrition amplifies results. Focus on a balanced diet rich in whole foods, lean proteins, and plenty of fruits and vegetables. Proper hydration is also crucial, as even mild dehydration can impair physical performance and slow metabolism.

Consider consulting a nutritionist to tailor a diet plan that complements your rucking regimen. Pay attention to your body's needs, ensuring you fuel adequately before a ruck and recover with nutritious foods afterward.

Rucking for Older Adults

Rucking offers numerous health benefits for older adults, promoting physical fitness, balance, and social engagement. Here's why rucking is an excellent choice for this population:

Improving Strength and Endurance

As we age, maintaining muscle mass and bone density becomes increasingly important. Rucking provides a low-impact strength workout that helps counteract age-related muscle loss. The added weight challenges muscles without the need for gym equipment, making it a convenient option for building strength.

Rucking also improves cardiovascular endurance. Regular aerobic exercise, like rucking, can enhance heart health, lower blood pressure, and improve overall endurance. By starting with short distances and lighter weights, older adults can gradually increase their stamina and enjoy the cardiovascular benefits of rucking.

Enhancing Balance and Coordination

Falls are a significant concern for older adults, often leading to injuries and decreased independence. Rucking helps improve balance and coordination by engaging core muscles and stabilizing muscles in the legs and hips. Walking on varied terrains, such as trails or grass, can further enhance proprioception and stability.

Incorporate balance exercises into your rucking routine, such as walking heel-to-toe or standing on one foot while rucking. These exercises can be done as part of a warm-up or cool-down to help improve balance over time.

Social Engagement and Mental Well-being

Rucking is not only a physical activity but also a social one. Joining a local rucking group or participating in organized rucking events can provide valuable social interaction and support. This social aspect is crucial for mental well-being, helping to reduce feelings of isolation and depression.

Rucking outdoors also offers mental health benefits. Nature has a calming effect, reducing stress and promoting relaxation. Encourage older adults to take advantage of parks, trails, and scenic routes for a refreshing and uplifting experience.

Family Rucking: Getting Kids Involved

Rucking is a family-friendly activity that encourages children to be active and explore the outdoors. Here's how to make rucking an enjoyable and educational experience for kids:

Making Rucking Fun and Engaging

For kids, the key to enjoying rucking is making it fun and adventurous. Plan routes with interesting landmarks, nature trails, or parks to keep children engaged. Turn the ruck into a treasure hunt or scavenger hunt, where kids can find and collect natural items like leaves or rocks.

Keep the pace manageable and include regular breaks for snacks and hydration. Short, frequent rucks are better suited for younger children, while older kids may enjoy longer distances and more challenging terrains.

Teaching Responsibility and Teamwork

Rucking with kids is an opportunity to teach them about responsibility and teamwork. Let them pack their own small backpacks with essentials like water, snacks, and a light jacket. Encourage them to take care of their belongings and look out for their siblings or friends during the ruck.

Working together as a family to plan routes, set goals, and achieve milestones can foster a sense of teamwork and accomplishment. Celebrate achievements, whether it's completing a new route or rucking a certain distance, to build confidence and motivation.

Instilling Healthy Habits

Introducing kids to rucking early on can instill lifelong healthy habits. Emphasize the importance of regular physical activity, outdoor exploration, and maintaining a balanced lifestyle. Discuss the benefits of exercise for physical and mental health, and encourage kids to set their own fitness goals.

Incorporating educational elements, such as learning about local wildlife or practicing mapreading skills, can make rucking a holistic and enriching experience for children.

Adapting Rucking for Different Fitness Levels

Rucking's versatility makes it accessible to individuals at various fitness levels, from beginners to seasoned athletes. Here's how to adapt rucking to meet different needs:

Beginners: Starting with the Basics

For those new to rucking, start with short distances and light weights to build a foundation of fitness. Focus on proper form and posture, keeping the core engaged and shoulders back. Begin with 15-20 minutes of rucking and gradually increase the duration and intensity as your fitness improves.

Track your progress by logging the distance, time, and weight carried. Set achievable goals, such as rucking twice a week, and celebrate small victories to stay motivated.

Intermediate: Building Endurance and Strength

Intermediate ruckers can challenge themselves by increasing the weight of their packs and incorporating varied terrains, such as hills or uneven trails. Incorporate interval training by alternating between brisk walking and slower paces to boost cardiovascular endurance.

Consider joining a rucking club or group to connect with others who share your interests. Group rucks can provide motivation and accountability, helping you stay committed to your fitness journey.

Advanced: Pushing Limits and Competing

Experienced ruckers looking to push their limits can participate in organized rucking events and competitions, such as GORUCK challenges. These events test physical and mental endurance, often involving long distances and team-based activities.

Advanced ruckers can also incorporate crosstraining, such as strength training, running, or cycling, to enhance overall fitness. Focus on specific goals, whether it's completing a marathon-length ruck or achieving a personal best in a competitive event.

Rucking for Special Populations

Rucking can be adapted to accommodate individuals with specific needs or limitations, making it an inclusive activity for all. Here's how to tailor rucking for special populations:

Individuals with Physical Disabilities

Rucking can be modified for individuals with physical disabilities, such as mobility impairments or chronic conditions. Focus on lighter weights and shorter distances, and choose accessible routes with smooth surfaces.

Consider using adaptive equipment, such as specialized backpacks or walking aids, to enhance comfort and safety. Always consult with a healthcare professional or fitness expert to ensure the rucking routine is appropriate and safe.

Rucking for Injury Recovery

Rucking can be a beneficial part of a rehabilitation program for individuals recovering from injuries. The low-impact nature of rucking allows for gradual reintroduction of physical activity, helping rebuild strength and endurance.

Start with minimal weight and short distances, focusing on proper form and alignment. Gradually increase the intensity and duration as recovery progresses. Collaborate with a physical therapist to develop a rucking plan that supports your rehabilitation goals.

Rucking for Mental Health and Well-being

Rucking offers mental health benefits, making it an effective tool for individuals seeking to improve their mental well-being. The combination of physical activity, outdoor exposure, and social interaction can reduce symptoms of anxiety and depression, boost mood, and enhance overall mental health.

Encourage individuals to practice mindfulness while rucking, focusing on the sights, sounds, and sensations of the environment. Incorporate breathing exercises and meditation techniques to promote relaxation and stress relief.

Tips for Safe and Enjoyable Rucking

To ensure a safe and enjoyable rucking experience for everyone, consider the following tips:

Choosing the Right Gear

Invest in a quality backpack with adjustable straps and padding for comfort. Select appropriate footwear that provides

support and traction, and dress in moisture-wicking clothing to prevent chafing and overheating.

Prioritizing Safety

Plan routes in advance, considering factors such as terrain, weather, and accessibility. Carry essentials like water, snacks, a map, and a first aid kit. Inform someone of your planned route and estimated return time, especially when rucking alone or in unfamiliar areas.

Listening to Your Body

Pay attention to your body's signals, such as fatigue, discomfort, or pain. Adjust the pace, weight, or distance as needed to prevent injury. Incorporate rest days into your routine to allow for recovery and avoid overtraining.

Staying Motivated

Set specific, measurable goals to stay motivated and track your progress. Consider joining a rucking community or group for support and camaraderie. Celebrate achievements and milestones to maintain enthusiasm and commitment.

Rucking for Weight Loss

Rucking is an effective and accessible exercise that combines the benefits of strength training and cardiovascular workouts. By simply walking with a weighted backpack, individuals can enhance their fitness routines and accelerate weight loss efforts.

Here's how rucking can be leveraged as a powerful tool for weight loss:

Enhanced Caloric Burn

Rucking increases caloric expenditure compared to regular walking because the added weight in the backpack increases the intensity of the exercise. This boost in intensity helps create a caloric deficit, which is essential for weight loss. The more weight carried, the more calories burned, making rucking an efficient way to enhance energy expenditure without requiring high-impact activities like running.

Low-Impact, Sustainable Exercise

Unlike high-impact workouts, rucking is low-impact and gentle on the joints, making it suitable for people of various fitness levels and ages. It can be easily incorporated into daily routines, such as commuting to work, walking the dog, or hiking on weekends. Its simplicity and adaptability make rucking a sustainable exercise option that can be maintained over the long term, supporting consistent weight loss efforts.

Building Muscle and Boosting Metabolism

Rucking engages major muscle groups, including the legs, core, and upper body. This engagement promotes muscle growth and maintenance, which is crucial for increasing metabolism. A higher resting metabolic rate means your body burns more calories at rest, supporting long-term weight management. As muscle mass increases, so does the body's ability to burn calories efficiently, even outside of exercise sessions.

Combining Rucking with Nutrition

For optimal weight loss results, pair rucking with a balanced diet. Focus on whole foods, lean proteins, healthy fats, and plenty of fruits and vegetables. Proper hydration is also crucial, as dehydration can impair physical performance and slow metabolism. By combining rucking with mindful nutrition, individuals can amplify their weight loss outcomes and promote overall health.

Tracking Progress and Setting Goals

Keep track of rucking sessions by logging distance, time, and weight carried. Setting specific, measurable goals helps maintain motivation and monitor progress. Celebrate milestones, such as reaching a new distance or carrying a heavier load, to stay inspired and committed to your weight loss journey.

Adapting Rucking for Older Adults

Rucking is an excellent exercise choice for older adults, offering a range of physical and mental health benefits. With its low-impact nature and adaptability, rucking can help older individuals maintain fitness, enhance balance, and enjoy social engagement.

Improving Physical Fitness

Rucking is a weight-bearing exercise that helps improve muscle strength, bone density, and cardiovascular health. By carrying a weighted backpack, older adults can build and maintain muscle mass, which is important for preventing agerelated muscle loss. Regular rucking also supports heart health and enhances endurance, contributing to overall physical fitness.

Enhancing Balance and Coordination

Rucking engages core and stabilizing muscles, which are essential for maintaining balance and coordination. This is particularly important for older adults, as improved balance can reduce the risk of falls and injuries. Walking on varied terrains, such as trails or grassy areas, further enhances proprioception and stability, making rucking a valuable tool for improving overall balance.

Promoting Mental Well-being and Social Interaction

Rucking offers mental health benefits by reducing stress, anxiety, and depression. Being outdoors and engaging in physical activity can boost mood and promote relaxation. Rucking with a group or partner provides valuable social interaction and support, reducing feelings of isolation and enhancing mental well-being.

Adapting Rucking for Individual Needs

Older adults should start with lighter weights and shorter distances, gradually increasing as their fitness level improves. Focus on proper form and posture to prevent injury and maximize benefits. Choose accessible routes that are safe and enjoyable, and incorporate regular breaks for rest and hydration. Consulting with a healthcare professional before starting a new exercise routine is recommended, especially for those with existing health conditions.

Family Rucking: Getting Kids Involved

Rucking is a family-friendly activity that encourages children to be active, explore the outdoors, and learn valuable life skills. Here's how to make rucking an enjoyable and educational experience for kids:

Making Rucking Fun and Engaging

For kids, the key to enjoying rucking is making it fun and adventurous. Plan routes with interesting landmarks, nature trails, or parks to keep children engaged. Turn the ruck into a treasure hunt or scavenger hunt, where kids can find and collect natural items like leaves or rocks. Incorporate games and challenges to keep them motivated and entertained.

Teaching Responsibility and Teamwork

Rucking with kids is an opportunity to teach them about responsibility and teamwork. Let them pack their own small backpacks with essentials like water, snacks, and a light jacket. Encourage them to take care of their belongings and look out for their siblings or friends during the ruck. Working together as a family to plan routes, set goals, and achieve milestones fosters a sense of teamwork and accomplishment.

Instilling Healthy Habits

Introducing kids to rucking early on can instill lifelong healthy habits. Emphasize the importance of regular physical activity, outdoor exploration, and maintaining a balanced lifestyle. Discuss the benefits of exercise for physical and mental health, and encourage kids to set their own fitness goals. Incorporating educational elements, such as learning about local wildlife or practicing mapreading skills, makes rucking a holistic and enriching experience for children.

Adjusting Rucking for Different Ages and Abilities

Tailor the rucking experience to the age and fitness level of the children involved. Younger kids may benefit from shorter distances and lighter weights, while older children might enjoy more challenging routes and heavier packs. Keep the pace manageable and include regular breaks for snacks and hydration. Be attentive to each child's needs and preferences to ensure a positive experience.

By adapting rucking for weight loss, older adults, and families, you can create a comprehensive guide that highlights the versatility and benefits of this accessible exercise. Rucking offers something for everyone, making it an ideal activity for individuals and families looking to improve their health and enjoy the great outdoors together.

CHAPTER 9

Mind Over Matter: The Mental Side of Rucking

Mind Over Matter: The Mental Side of Rucking

Rucking, while a physical endeavor, is equally a mental challenge. The adage "mind over matter" rings particularly true in this context.

The Mental Grind

- **Overcoming discomfort:** The physical strain of carrying weight for extended periods can be mentally taxing. Overcoming the urge to quit is as crucial as physical endurance.
- **Building mental resilience:** Rucking pushes mental boundaries, helping individuals develop perseverance and determination.
- **Focus and concentration:** Maintaining focus on the task at hand, especially during long rucks, is vital for mental clarity.
- **Goal setting:** Setting clear and achievable goals can provide a mental roadmap and motivation.

Mental Strategies

- **Visualization:** Imagining successful completion of a ruck can boost motivation.
- **Positive self-talk:** Encouraging words can counteract negative thoughts.
- **Mindfulness:** Focusing on the present moment can help manage discomfort.
- **Breaking it down:** Dividing the ruck into smaller segments can make the challenge seem less daunting.

The Reward

Overcoming mental challenges during rucking leads to:

- Increased self-confidence
- Improved problem-solving skills
- Enhanced mental toughness
- A greater sense of accomplishment

Remember, the mind is a powerful tool. By training it alongside the body, you can unlock your full potential as a ruck marcher.

Mental Preparation for Rucking Challenges

Rucking challenges, such as long-distance hikes or obstacle course races, demand exceptional mental fortitude. Here are some strategies to fortify your mind:

Pre-Ruck Mental Preparation

- **Goal Setting:** Clearly define your goals, whether it's finishing the ruck, maintaining a specific pace, or simply enjoying the experience.
- **Visualization:** Imagine yourself successfully completing the challenge. Visualize overcoming obstacles and reaching your goals.
- **Positive Affirmations:** Replace negative thoughts with positive affirmations. Remind yourself of your capabilities and reasons for undertaking the challenge.
- **Physical and Mental Conditioning:** Ensure you're physically prepared. A wellconditioned body boosts mental resilience. Cross-training with activities like yoga or meditation can enhance mental focus.

During the Ruck: Overcoming Challenges

- **Breaking it Down:** Divide the ruck into smaller, manageable segments. Focusing on completing each segment can help prevent overwhelm.

- **Mindfulness Techniques:** Practice deep breathing and mindfulness to stay centered and focused.
- **Positive Self-Talk:** Continuously remind yourself of your strength and determination.

- **Find a Rhythm:** Develop a consistent pace and rhythm to maintain mental and physical equilibrium.
- **Leverage the Group:** If rucking with a team, mutual support can be a powerful motivator.

Post-Ruck Reflection

- **Analyze Performance:** Reflect on what went well and areas for improvement.
- **Reward Yourself:** Acknowledge your accomplishments, no matter how small.
- **Learn and Grow:** Use the experience to build mental resilience for future challenges.

Types of Rucking Challenges and Overcoming Them

Rucking, while rewarding, can present various challenges. Here are some common ones and strategies to overcome them:

Physical Challenges

- **Fatigue:**
  - Pace yourself: Avoid starting too fast. o Short breaks: Take short rest periods to recover. o Proper nutrition: Fuel your body with energy-rich foods.

- **Muscle Soreness:**
  - Gradual increase: Build up the weight and distance gradually.
  - Stretching: Incorporate stretching before and after rucks.
  - Cross-training: Complement rucking with other activities like swimming or cycling.
- **Foot and Blister Issues:**
  - Proper footwear: Invest in quality, wellfitting boots or shoes.
  - Moisture management: Use moisturewicking socks and consider antichafing products. o Regular checks: Inspect your feet during breaks.

Mental Challenges

- **Boredom:**

  - Vary routes: Explore different terrains and environments.

o Podcasts or audiobooks: Keep your mind engaged. o Rucking buddy: Social interaction can make the time pass faster.

- **Doubt and Fear:**
  - o Positive self-talk: Remind yourself of your capabilities. o Break it down: Focus on smaller goals within the larger challenge.
  - o Visualization: Imagine yourself successfully completing the ruck.
- **Physical and Mental Fatigue:**
  - o Pace yourself: Avoid pushing too hard too soon.
  - o Short breaks: Take short rest periods to recover.
  - o Positive reinforcement: Reward yourself for reaching milestones.

Environmental Challenges

- **Weather:**
  - o Proper gear: Dress appropriately for the weather conditions.
  - o Hydration: Drink plenty of fluids, especially in hot weather. o Sun protection: Wear sunscreen, a hat, and sunglasses. • **Terrain:**
  - o Varying pace: Adjust your pace based on the terrain.

   ○ Proper footwear: Wear shoes with good traction. ○ Focus on footing: Pay attention to where you place your feet.

By understanding these challenges and implementing appropriate strategies, you can enhance your rucking experience and increase your chances of success.

Building Mental Resilience: A Cornerstone of Well-being

Mental resilience is the ability to adapt and bounce back from adversity.

It's about finding strength in challenges, learning from setbacks, and emerging stronger. While it's a skill that can be developed, it's also influenced by factors like genetics, life experiences, and support systems.

Understanding Mental Resilience

Resilience is not about being invincible or never experiencing difficulties. Instead, it's about how we respond to challenges. Resilient individuals possess a unique combination of qualities, including:

- **Optimism:** A positive outlook can help individuals see challenges as opportunities for growth.
- **Adaptability:** The ability to adjust to change and find new ways to cope.
- **Problem-solving:** Effective problem-solving skills help navigate through difficulties.
- **Self-awareness:** Understanding one's emotions and strengths is crucial for building resilience.
- **Strong support system:** A network of supportive friends and family can provide encouragement and assistance.

Developing Mental Resilience

Building mental resilience is a journey, not a destination. Here are some strategies to foster it:

Cultivate a Growth Mindset

- **Embrace challenges:** View obstacles as opportunities for learning and growth.
- **Believe in your abilities:** Develop a strong sense of self-efficacy.

-

- **Learn from setbacks:** Analyze failures to identify lessons and improve future performance.

  Seek feedback: Constructive criticism can help identify areas for improvement.

Build Strong Relationships

- **Nurture connections:** Spend quality time with loved ones.
- **Seek support:** Don't hesitate to ask for help when needed.
- **Join groups:** Connect with people who share similar interests.

Practice Self-Care

- **Prioritize sleep:** Adequate rest is essential for mental and physical well-being.
- **Manage stress:** Incorporate relaxation techniques like meditation or yoga.
- **Exercise regularly:** Physical activity boosts mood and energy levels.
- **Maintain a healthy diet:** Nourish your body for optimal brain function.

•

Develop Coping Mechanisms

- **Problem-solving:** Break down challenges into smaller, manageable steps.

  Time management: Effective time management reduces stress.
- **Humor:** Find ways to laugh and see the lighter side of life.
- **Mindfulness:** Focus on the present moment to reduce anxiety.

Learn from Adversity

- **Identify strengths:** Reflect on how you've overcome challenges in the past.
- **Develop a positive outlook:** Focus on what you can control rather than what you can't.
- **Seek professional help if needed:** Therapists can provide tools and support.

-

Resilience in Different Life Stages

Building resilience is a lifelong process. Children, adolescents, adults, and older adults face unique challenges. Tailoring resilience strategies to each stage is crucial.

- **Children:** Foster a sense of security, encourage problem-solving, and teach emotional regulation.
- **Adolescents:** Promote independence, build self-esteem, and provide support networks.

  Adults: Encourage work-life balance, stress management, and continuous learning.
- **Older adults:** Maintain social connections, find purpose, and adapt to changes.

Resilience in the Workplace

Resilience is essential for navigating workplace challenges. Organizations can foster a resilient culture by:

- **Supporting employee well-being:** Offering resources for stress management and mental health.

-
- **Encouraging work-life balance:** Promoting healthy boundaries and time off.
- **Providing opportunities for growth:**
  Offering training and development programs.
- **Building a supportive work environment:** Fostering open communication and collaboration.

Conclusion

Building mental resilience is a journey that requires ongoing effort and self-awareness. By incorporating the strategies outlined above, individuals can enhance their ability to cope with challenges, thrive under pressure, and experience greater overall wellbeing. Remember, resilience is not about avoiding difficulties but about overcoming them with strength and determination.

Personal stories of transformation

Story 1: From Couch Potato to Conqueror

I was the epitome of a couch potato. My world revolved around the TV screen, fast food, and endless scrolling through social media. I was physically and mentally stagnant, a prisoner of my own comfort zone. My weight crept up, my selfesteem plummeted, and I felt a growing sense of despair.

Then came the day a friend introduced me to rucking. The idea of carrying a weighted backpack and walking seemed absurd. But desperation had a way of making the impossible seem achievable. I started small, with a light pack and short distances. The initial struggle was immense. My body ached, my mind protested, and I was tempted to quit countless times.

Yet, something about the rhythm of my footsteps and the weight on my shoulders was strangely addictive. With each step, I felt a sense of accomplishment.

The physical exertion cleared my mind, and the solitude of the open road provided a much-needed escape. Gradually, the walks became longer, the weight heavier, and the challenges more demanding.

The physical transformation was evident. My body toned, my stamina increased, and the number on the scale started to drop. But the most profound changes happened within. The once-timid and insecure individual began to discover a strength and resilience he never knew existed. The fear of failure was replaced by a determination to succeed.

Rucking became more than just exercise; it was a metaphor for life. Every uphill climb, every obstacle encountered, was a reflection of the challenges we face in our daily lives. And with each victory, my confidence grew.

One day, I found myself signing up for a 50-mile rucking challenge. The idea was terrifying, but the thought of quitting was even more so. Training was grueling, both physically and mentally. There were moments of doubt, when the weight of the backpack seemed to crush my spirit. But I pushed through, drawing strength from the countless hours spent on the road.

The day of the challenge arrived. The initial excitement was soon replaced by a wave of nerves. As I set off, I focused on one step at a time, one mile at a time. The journey was arduous, filled with pain and exhaustion. But with each step, I felt a surge of accomplishment.

When I finally crossed the finish line, the sense of achievement was overwhelming. I had conquered not just the physical challenge, but also the mental demons that had held me back for so long. Rucking had transformed me from a sedentary, self-doubting individual into a confident, resilient person.

The journey continues, and the challenges never truly end. But with each step, I am reminded of the strength I have discovered within myself. Rucking is more than just a physical activity; it's a way of life, a testament to the human spirit's ability to overcome adversity.

Story 2: Finding Purpose Through Rucking

Sarah was a successful career woman, juggling a demanding job with the pressures of modern life. She had everything on the surface - a thriving career, a loving family, and a comfortable lifestyle. Yet, a nagging emptiness persisted. She felt disconnected, unfulfilled, and trapped in a routine that was devoid of meaning.

Seeking an escape, Sarah stumbled upon the world of rucking. Initially drawn to the physical challenge, she soon discovered a deeper connection to herself and the world around her. The solitary nature of rucking provided a much-needed respite from the constant noise and demands of her daily life.

As she ventured into nature, carrying the weight of her backpack, she found a sense of grounding. The rhythmic motion of her steps became a meditative practice, allowing her mind to wander and find clarity. The physical exertion cleared the mental fog, and she began to see life with a renewed perspective.

Rucking became a catalyst for personal growth. The challenges she faced on the trail mirrored the obstacles she encountered in her professional and personal life. With each step, she developed resilience, determination, and a stronger sense of self. The weight on her back became a metaphor for the burdens she carried, and with each mile, she felt lighter, freer.

Through rucking, Sarah rediscovered her passion for helping others. Inspired by her own transformation, she started a local rucking group to encourage others to embrace the physical and mental benefits of this unique exercise. She became a mentor, a friend, and a source of inspiration for countless individuals.

Her newfound purpose brought a sense of fulfillment that had been missing from her life. She realized that true happiness comes from serving others and making a positive impact on the world. Rucking had not only transformed her physically but had also awakened her soul.

Story 3: A Soldier's Journey: Rucking for Recovery

For Sergeant Johnathan, the physical and mental scars of war ran deep. After multiple deployments, he struggled with PTSD, chronic pain, and a profound sense of isolation. The transition to civilian life was a daunting challenge, and he found himself lost and adrift.

Desperate for a way to reclaim his life, Johnathan turned to rucking. The familiar weight on his back felt like a comforting embrace. The rhythmic motion of walking provided a sense of grounding and purpose. As he ventured into nature, he found solace in the solitude.

Initially, the physical demands were overwhelming. The pain was a constant companion, and the mental anguish often threatened to consume him. But with each step, he pushed through the discomfort, drawing strength from his military training.

Rucking became a form of therapy. The physical exertion helped to alleviate the symptoms of PTSD, while the mental challenge forced him to confront his demons. The solitude of the trail provided a safe space to process his emotions and find a sense of peace.

As his physical strength returned, so too did his mental resilience. The camaraderie of fellow ruckers provided a much-needed support system. Together, they shared stories, offered encouragement, and found healing in the shared experience.

Johnathan's journey was not without setbacks. There were days when the pain was unbearable, and the memories of war threatened to consume him. But through perseverance and determination, he found a way to overcome these challenges.

Rucking became a symbol of his resilience. The weight on his back represented the burdens he carried, and with each step, he was shedding those burdens, one by one. The journey was long and arduous, but the rewards were immeasurable. Johnathan had found a path to healing, a sense of purpose, and a renewed appreciation for life

These are true life stories and I want you to pick inspiration from them.

The Community Connection: Finding Support Through Rucking

While individual journeys are essential, the power of community cannot be overstated. Rucking, inherently a solitary activity, can be transformed into a shared experience, fostering a sense of belonging and mutual support.

The Importance of Community in Rucking

- **Shared Experiences:** Bonding over shared challenges and triumphs strengthens connections.
- **Motivation and Support:** Encouragement from fellow ruckers can be a game-changer.
- **Knowledge Sharing:** Learning from others' experiences can enhance one's rucking journey.
- **Accountability:** Committing to group rucks can increase consistency.

Building a Supportive Rucking Community

- **Online Platforms:** Utilize social media and online forums to connect with like-minded individuals.
- **Local Rucking Groups:** Organize in-person meetups to foster stronger bonds.
- **Mentorship Programs:** Pair experienced ruckers with newcomers.
- **Shared Goals:** Create group challenges or events to work towards common objectives.

Overcoming Challenges in Building Community

- **Diversity and Inclusion:** Ensure the community is welcoming to all backgrounds and fitness levels.
- **Geographical Limitations:** Utilize technology to connect with remote members.
- **Balancing Individual and Group Goals:** Respect individual needs while fostering a sense of community.

The Impact of Community on Rucking Success

A strong rucking community can significantly impact an individual's journey:

- **Increased Motivation:** Shared goals and support can drive persistence.

- **Improved Mental Health:** Social connection reduces feelings of isolation.
- **Enhanced Performance:** Learning from others can lead to better techniques and results.
- **Lifelong Friendships:** Strong bonds formed through shared experiences.

By fostering a sense of community, rucking can become more than just a physical activity; it can be a transformative experience that enriches lives.

CHAPTER 10

Resources and Communities

Rucking and Community: A Shared Journey

While the physical act of rucking is a solitary endeavor, the shared experience can foster a powerful sense of community. Let's explore how rucking can bring people together and create a supportive network.

The Power of Shared Experience

Rucking, at its core, is a challenging activity. Sharing this experience with others creates a unique bond. The shared struggle, triumphs, and camaraderie forged on the trail can be incredibly powerful.

- **Shared Goals:** Whether it's weight loss, mental health, or physical fitness, a common goal can unite people.
- **Mutual Support:** Encouragement and support from fellow ruckers can be invaluable, especially during challenging times.
- **Sense of Belonging:** Being part of a rucking community provides a sense of belonging and connection.

Rucking as a Catalyst for Change

Rucking can be a catalyst for personal and community transformation.

- **Inspiring Others:** Sharing personal stories of transformation can motivate others to embark on their own rucking journeys.
- **Creating Support Networks:** Establishing local rucking groups can provide a platform for individuals to connect and support each other.
- **Giving Back:** Rucking can be used as a platform for fundraising or volunteering for charitable causes.

Challenges and Opportunities

While building a rucking community is rewarding, it also comes with challenges.

- **Balancing Individual Goals and Group Dynamics:** Ensuring everyone feels included and supported while maintaining individual objectives.
- **Overcoming Logistics:** Coordinating schedules, locations, and equipment can be time-consuming.
- **Maintaining Momentum:** Keeping the group engaged and motivated over time.

Despite these challenges, the potential benefits of a strong rucking community are immense. It can provide a supportive environment for personal growth, foster friendships, and create a positive impact on the community.

Building a Rucking Community: A Shared Journey

Types of Rucking Communities

Rucking communities can take various forms, each offering unique benefits:

- **Local Rucking Groups:**
    - **Benefits:** Strong sense of community, regular meet-ups, shared local knowledge.
    - **Challenges:** Can be limited by geographic location and group size.
- **Online Rucking Communities:**
    - **Benefits:** Global reach, diverse perspectives, 24/7 support.
    - **Challenges:** Lack of in-person connection, potential for online disengagement.
- **Military and Veteran Rucking Groups:**
    - **Benefits:** Shared experiences, camaraderie, support network.

- **Challenges:** Specific focus on military-related challenges and experiences.
- **Fitness-Based Rucking Groups:**
  - **Benefits:** Focus on physical fitness goals, variety of fitness levels.
  - **Challenges:** Potential for competition and comparison.

Building a Strong Rucking Community

Creating a thriving rucking community requires careful planning and execution.

- **Define Your Community's Purpose:** Clearly articulate the goals and values of your group.
- **Leverage Social Media:** Utilize platforms like Facebook, Instagram, and online forums to connect with potential members.
- **Organize Regular Events:** Plan group rucks, challenges, and social gatherings.
- **Foster Inclusivity:** Create a welcoming environment for all fitness levels and backgrounds.
- **Encourage Sharing:** Promote storytelling and sharing of experiences.
- **Give Back:** Participate in community service or fundraising initiatives.

Case Study: A Successful Rucking Community

The Midnight Ruckers, a group based in a bustling metropolis, exemplify the power of community. Founded by a group of friends passionate about rucking, they quickly grew into a thriving community. By organizing regular city-wide rucks, fitness challenges, and social events, they created a strong sense of belonging among members. Their commitment to giving back through volunteer work and fundraising initiatives further solidified their position as a positive force in the community.

Overcoming Challenges

Building a lasting community requires addressing potential challenges:

- **Maintaining Interest:** Continuously introduce new elements to keep members engaged.
- **Managing Growth:** Develop systems for managing increasing membership numbers.
- **Handling Conflicts:** Establish clear guidelines for resolving disagreements.

Technology and Community Building in Rucking

Technology has revolutionized how we connect and interact, and the rucking community is no exception.

Let's explore how technology can be leveraged to build and strengthen rucking communities.

Leveraging Technology for Community Building

- **Social Media Platforms:**
  - Creating a strong online presence can attract potential members. ○ Sharing photos, videos, and stories can inspire and engage the community.
  - Utilizing groups and forums for discussions and event planning.
- **Fitness Tracking Apps:**
  - Integrating with fitness trackers can gamify the rucking experience. ○ Sharing achievements and progress can motivate members. ○ Tracking metrics can help individuals set goals and monitor improvement.
- **Online Rucking Challenges:**
  - Creating virtual challenges can foster competition and camaraderie.
  - Offering prizes or rewards can increase participation.
- **Virtual Rucking:**
  - Connecting with people from different locations through online platforms. ○ Offering virtual training sessions and support groups.

Retaining Members in a Digital Age

- **Personalized Experiences:** Offering tailored content and challenges based on individual preferences.
- **Strong Community Focus:** Prioritizing member interactions and support.
- **Offline Events:** Balancing online engagement with in-person meetups.
- **Continuous Improvement:** Regularly seeking feedback and adapting to members' needs.

Challenges and Opportunities

While technology offers numerous benefits, it also presents challenges:

- **Screen Time vs. Outdoor Engagement:** Balancing virtual interactions with real-world connections.
- **Data Privacy:** Protecting members' personal information.
- **Maintaining Authenticity:** Ensuring genuine connections in a digital world.

Balancing Online and Offline Engagement in

Rucking Communities

The digital age presents both opportunities and challenges for building and maintaining strong rucking communities. Striking a balance between online and offline interactions is crucial for fostering a sense of belonging and connection.

Leveraging Technology for Offline Engagement

Technology can be a powerful tool for enhancing inperson experiences.

- **Event Planning and Coordination:** Utilize online platforms to organize group rucks, challenges, and social events.

- **Communication Tools:** Create group chats or messaging platforms for real-time updates and discussions.
- **Fitness Tracking Integration:** Encourage members to share their progress and achievements to inspire others.

Overcoming Challenges of Online Engagement

- **Encouraging Real-World Interactions:** Organize regular in-person meetups to complement online connections.
- **Building Trust:** Foster a sense of authenticity and trust through open communication.
- **Preventing Isolation:** Encourage members to engage in offline activities together.

Case Study: A Hybrid Approach

A successful rucking community might combine the best of both worlds:

- **Online Platform:** A dedicated website or app for member profiles, event calendars, forums, and fitness tracking.
- **Local Chapters:** Establishing regional groups for in-person meetups and events.
- **Hybrid Events:** Organizing events that combine virtual and in-person elements, such

as virtual challenges with local meetups for celebrations.

By carefully considering the strengths and weaknesses of both online and offline engagement, rucking communities can create a dynamic and fulfilling experience for their members.

Measuring the Impact of Online and Offline Engagement

Understanding the impact of your communitybuilding efforts is crucial for making data-driven decisions. By tracking key metrics, you can measure the effectiveness of your strategies and identify areas for improvement.

Key Performance Indicators (KPIs)

- **Membership Growth:** Track the number of new members joining the community.
- **Member Engagement:** Measure the frequency of member participation in online and offline activities.
- **Social Media Metrics:** Analyze follower growth, engagement rates, and reach on various platforms.
- **Event Attendance:** Track the number of attendees at in-person events.

•

- **Member Satisfaction:** Conduct surveys or polls to gauge member satisfaction.

Case Studies of Successful Hybrid Communities
The Rucking Ramblers: This group effectively combines online and offline engagement by offering virtual challenges, online support forums, and regular in-person meetups. They track membership growth, event attendance, and social media engagement to measure their impact.

- **The Urban Hikers:** This city-based community focuses on creating a strong sense of belonging through in-person events while leveraging online platforms for communication and event planning. They measure member satisfaction through surveys and track event attendance to gauge engagement.

Strategies for Data Collection and Analysis

- **Utilize Social Media Analytics:** Most platforms offer insights into audience demographics, engagement, and post performance.
- **Conduct Surveys and Questionnaires:** Gather feedback from members about their experience and satisfaction.

- **Track Event Attendance:** Use sign-up sheets or event registration platforms to monitor attendance.
- **Analyze Fitness Tracker Data:** If applicable, collect and analyze data on members' activity levels.

Tools and Platforms for Data Collection and Analysis in Rucking Communities

To effectively measure the impact of your rucking community, utilizing the right tools is essential. Here are some options:

Data Collection Tools

- **Social Media Analytics:** Most platforms offer built-in analytics to track engagement, reach, and demographics.
- **Survey and Poll Platforms:** Tools like SurveyMonkey, Google Forms, or Typeform can be used to gather feedback from members.
- **Event Registration Platforms:** Platforms like Eventbrite or Meetup can track attendee information and provide analytics.
- **Fitness Tracker Integration:** If your community utilizes fitness trackers, consider integrating data for analysis.

-

Data Analysis Tools

- **Spreadsheet Software:** Tools like Excel or Google Sheets can be used for basic data analysis and visualization.
- **Data Visualization Tools:** Platforms like Tableau or Power BI can create interactive dashboards for complex data sets.

  Social Media Analytics Tools: Some social media platforms offer advanced analytics tools for in-depth analysis.

Gamification to Boost Engagement

Gamification can make community participation more fun and rewarding.

- **Point Systems:** Reward members for participating in activities, reaching milestones, or inviting friends.
- **Badges and Achievements:** Recognize member accomplishments with virtual rewards.
- **Leaderboards:** Create friendly competition to motivate members.
- **Challenges and Contests:** Organize themed challenges or competitions to encourage participation.

By combining data collection, analysis, and gamification, rucking communities can gain valuable insights into member behavior, preferences, and overall satisfaction. This information can be used to refine strategies, improve member experiences, and foster a thriving community.

Gamification and Member Retention in Rucking Communities

Gamification can be a powerful tool for increasing member engagement and retention in rucking communities. By incorporating game-like elements, you can make the experience more fun, rewarding, and competitive.

Gamification Strategies

- **Point-Based Systems:** Award points for various activities like attending events, completing challenges, or recruiting new members.
- **Leaderboards:** Create leaderboards for different categories such as distance covered, weight carried, or number of events attended.
- **Badges and Achievements:** Recognize member accomplishments with virtual badges or awards.

-
- **Challenges and Competitions:** Organize themed challenges or competitions to encourage participation.
- **Tiered Rewards:** Offer different levels of rewards based on points or achievements.

Examples of Gamification in Action

- **The Rucking Rally:** A monthly challenge where members compete to cover the most distance or climb the most elevation.

  The Rucking Rookie: A program for new members with a structured point system to encourage participation and goal setting.
- **The Rucking Ambassador:** A recognition program for members who actively recruit new members and contribute to the community.

Maintaining Member Engagement Over Time

- **Diverse Activities:** Offer a variety of activities to cater to different interests and fitness levels.
- **Regular Communication:** Keep members informed about upcoming events, challenges, and community updates.

- **Personalized Experiences:** Tailor content and recommendations based on member preferences.
- **Feedback Loop:** Continuously seek feedback from members to improve the community experience.
- **Celebrate Achievements:** Recognize and celebrate member milestones and successes.

Case Studies of Successful Gamification in Rucking Communities

To illustrate the power of gamification, let's examine a few successful case studies:

Case Study 1: The Rucking Rally

- **Gamification Elements:** A monthly competition with points awarded based on distance covered, elevation gained, and group participation.
- **Impact:** Increased member engagement, friendly competition, and a sense of camaraderie.
- **Lessons Learned:** Clear and transparent rules, regular communication, and offering various challenges to cater to different fitness levels are essential.

Case Study 2: The Rucking Rookie Program

- **Gamification Elements:** A tiered system with rewards for completing specific milestones, such as attending a certain number of rucks or covering a set distance.
- **Impact:** Improved retention for new members, a sense of accomplishment, and a clear path for progression.
- **Lessons Learned:** Providing regular support and encouragement is crucial for new members. Offering a variety of challenges helps to keep them engaged.

Measuring the Impact of Gamification

To assess the effectiveness of gamification strategies, consider these metrics:

- **Increased member engagement:** Measure participation rates in gamified activities.
- **Retention rates:** Track member retention before and after implementing gamification.
- **Social media engagement:** Analyze how gamification impacts social media interactions.
- **Member satisfaction:** Conduct surveys to gauge members' perceptions of gamification.

By tracking these metrics, you can determine the ROI of your gamification efforts and make adjustments as needed.

Tools and Platforms for Gamification in Rucking Communities

To effectively implement gamification strategies, consider these tools and platforms:

Dedicated Gamification Platforms

While many general-purpose platforms can be adapted, dedicated gamification platforms offer specific features tailored to this purpose.

- **StriveCloud:** Provides a comprehensive suite of tools for creating gamified experiences.
- **Badgeville:** Offers a platform for building loyalty programs and gamified experiences.

- **Bunchball:** Provides a range of gamification elements for motivating user behavior.

Social Media and Community Platforms

Existing social media platforms can be leveraged for gamification:

- **Facebook Groups:** Create groups for sharing achievements, challenges, and support.
- **Instagram:** Utilize stories, reels, and challenges to engage members.
- **Strava:** Connect with fitness-focused communities and track progress.

Fitness Tracking Apps

Integrate with fitness tracking apps to gamify the rucking experience:

- **Strava:** Offers challenges, segments, and leaderboards.
- **Fitbit:** Provides step challenges and badges.
- **Apple Health:** Integrates with various apps for tracking and sharing data.

Custom-Built Solutions

For complex gamification systems, consider developing a custom platform:

Benefits: Tailored to specific needs, full control over features.
- **Challenges:** Requires technical expertise and development resources.

Preventing Burnout from Excessive Gamification

While gamification can be highly effective, it's essential to avoid overdoing it.

- **Balance:** Combine gamification with genuine community building and shared experiences.
- **Variety:** Offer a mix of gamified and nongamified activities.
- **Player Choice:** Allow members to opt out of gamified elements if desired.
- **Real-World Rewards:** Consider offering tangible rewards in addition to virtual ones.

By carefully selecting and implementing the right tools and strategies, rucking communities can create engaging and rewarding experiences for their members while preventing burnout.

Gamification Ideas for Different Types of

Rucking Communities

Gamification can be tailored to specific types of rucking communities to enhance engagement and motivation. Let's explore some ideas:

Fitness-Focused Rucking Communities

- **Step Challenges:** Encourage members to reach daily, weekly, or monthly step goals.
- **Weight Challenge:** Promote gradual weight increase for those aiming to build strength.
- **Time Trials:** Organize timed rucking events to foster competition and improvement.

Mental Health and Wellness-Focused Rucking

Communities

- **Mindfulness Challenges:** Encourage members to focus on mental well-being through challenges like meditation or journaling.
- **Support Badge:** Award badges for providing support and encouragement to fellow members.
- **Progress Journaling:** Promote reflection and personal growth through journaling challenges.

Adventure-Focused Rucking Communities

- **Explore Challenges:** Encourage members to discover new trails or locations.
- **Photography Contest:** Promote sharing beautiful scenery and capturing the spirit of adventure.

    Navigation Challenge: Test members' navigation skills with map and compass challenges.

Military and Veteran Rucking Communities

- **Challenge Coins:** Award coins for completing specific challenges or milestones.
- **Team Competitions:** Foster camaraderie and competition through team-based challenges.
- **Virtual Rucking Rallies:** Connect members from different locations for shared experiences.

Measuring the Impact of Gamification on

Member Retention

To assess the effectiveness of gamification strategies, consider these key metrics:

- •
  - **Increased participation:** Track the number of members participating in gamified activities.
  - **Retention rates:** Compare member retention before and after implementing gamification.
  - **Member satisfaction:** Conduct surveys to measure how gamification impacts overall satisfaction.
  - **Social media engagement:** Analyze how gamification influences social media interactions.
  - **Qualitative feedback:** Gather insights through member testimonials and feedback.

Finding Local Rucking Groups

Finding Local Rucking Groups

Connecting with fellow ruckers in your area can significantly enhance your experience. Here are some strategies to find local groups:

- **Leverage Social Media:** Platforms like Facebook, Instagram, and Meetup are excellent resources for finding local rucking groups or creating your own. Use relevant hashtags to connect with potential members.

- **Check Local Gyms and Fitness Centers:** Many gyms and fitness centers offer outdoor group workouts or have community boards where you can post about your interest in rucking.
- **Explore Outdoor Recreation Stores:** These stores often have community bulletin boards or can provide information on local hiking or outdoor groups.
- **Attend Local Events:** Participate in community events like 5Ks, trail races, or

outdoor festivals to meet like-minded individuals.
- **Word of Mouth:** Spread the word among friends, family, and coworkers about your interest in rucking.

Online Resources and Communities

Online Resources and Communities

If you're unable to find a local group or prefer the flexibility of online connections, consider these options:

- **Rucking Forums and Online Communities:** Participate in online forums and social media groups dedicated to rucking.
- **Virtual Rucking Challenges:** Join online challenges to connect with ruckers worldwide.
- **Online Coaching and Support:** Consider hiring a virtual rucking coach or joining online support groups.

Recommended Reading and Further Exploration

Recommended Reading and Further Exploration
To deepen your understanding of rucking and its benefits, consider exploring these resources:

- **Books:** "The Rucking Handbook" by Travis k. Bone offers comprehensive information on rucking techniques, gear, and training.
- **Online Articles and Blogs:** Numerous websites and blogs provide valuable insights, tips, and inspiration.
- **Podcasts:** Listen to podcasts featuring rucking experts and interviews with experienced ruckers.
- **Documentaries:** Explore documentaries related to endurance sports or military training for additional motivation.

By combining these approaches, you can effectively find a rucking community that aligns with your goals and preferences, enhancing your overall experience and enjoyment of the sport.

CONCLUSION

Over the course of this comprehensive discussion, we delved into various facets of rucking, a unique and demanding physical activity that has gained popularity due to its blend of cardiovascular and strength training benefits. The exploration spanned from basic understanding and getting started to advanced techniques and preparation for competitions. This in-depth conclusion aims to encapsulate the wealth of information shared, providing a cohesive overview of rucking, its benefits, and how to excel in it.

Understanding Rucking

Rucking is essentially walking or hiking with a weighted rucksack. It originated from military training, where soldiers would carry heavy loads over long distances. This practice has transitioned into civilian fitness regimes, offering an accessible yet challenging workout that combines cardio and strength training.

Key Benefits

- **Full-Body Workout:** Rucking engages multiple muscle groups, including the back, shoulders, legs, and core.

- **Cardiovascular Health:** It enhances cardiovascular fitness by raising the heart rate over prolonged periods.
- **Mental Resilience:** The physical challenge promotes mental toughness and resilience.
- **Social Activity:** Often done in groups, rucking fosters camaraderie and community.
- **Accessible and Flexible:** It can be done virtually anywhere, with adjustable weights to suit different fitness levels.

Getting Started with Rucking

For beginners, starting with rucking involves understanding the basics and gradually building up the intensity.

Initial Steps

- **Choosing the Right Gear:** Invest in a good rucksack, sturdy footwear, and moisture-wicking clothing. Budget-friendly options are available for beginners.
- **Starting Light:** Begin with a lighter weight, around 10-20% of your body weight, and gradually increase as your strength and endurance improve.
- **Building a Routine:** Incorporate rucking into your weekly routine, starting with short distances and progressively increasing both the distance and weight.

Essential Gear

- **Backpack:** Ensure it is comfortable, durable, and has good weight distribution.
- **Footwear:** Choose shoes or boots that provide support and comfort. For different budgets, options range from basic hiking boots to specialized rucking shoes.
- **Clothing:** Moisture-wicking, breathable materials are ideal to prevent chafing and manage sweat.

First Aid Kit

- **Bandages and Blister Pads:** Essential for treating blisters and minor injuries.
- **Antiseptic Wipes:** For cleaning wounds.
- **Pain Relief Medication:** For muscle aches and pains.
- **Hydration Supplies:** Electrolyte tablets or powders to maintain hydration levels.

Mastering Rucking Techniques

Perfecting your technique is crucial for efficiency and injury prevention.

Proper Posture and Form

- **Straight Back:** Maintain a neutral spine to avoid strain.

-
  - **Engaged Core:** Keep your core tight to support the lower back.
  - **Arm Swing:** A natural arm swing helps with balance and momentum.
    Foot Placement: Aim for a heel-to-toe roll to reduce impact on the joints.

Efficient Breathing Techniques

- **Rhythmic Breathing:** Match your breath with your steps to maintain a steady pace.
- **Deep Breathing:** Engage the diaphragm to maximize oxygen intake and reduce fatigue.

Pacing and Cadence

- **Steady Pace:** Find a pace that you can sustain over long distances without burning out.
- **Cadence Control:** Maintain a consistent cadence to improve efficiency and reduce the risk of injury.

Navigating Different Terrains

- **Uphill:** Lean slightly forward, take shorter steps, and use your arms for balance.
- **Downhill:** Lean back slightly, keep your steps controlled, and use your core for stability.
- **Uneven Terrain:** Pay close attention to foot placement to avoid tripping or slipping.

Incorporating Strength Training

- **Supplementary Exercises:** Include squats, lunges, and deadlifts in your routine to build leg and core strength.
  Functional Movements: Practice exercises that mimic the movements used in rucking.

Hydration and Nutrition

- **Hydration:** Drink water regularly, and use electrolyte supplements if necessary.
- **Pre-Ruck Nutrition:** Consume a balanced meal with carbohydrates, protein, and fats to fuel your body.
- **During Ruck Nutrition:** Carry easily digestible snacks like energy bars or gels.

Interval Training

- **High-Intensity Intervals:** Incorporate bursts of highintensity rucking followed by recovery periods to boost endurance.
- **Hill Intervals:** Ruck up and down hills to improve strength and cardiovascular fitness.

Monitoring Progress

- **Track Metrics:** Use a fitness tracker or app to monitor distance, pace, and elevation.
- **Set Goals:** Establish short-term and long-term goals to stay motivated and measure progress.

Safety First: Essential Tips for New Ruckers

Safety is paramount in rucking to prevent injuries and ensure a positive experience.

Gradual Progression

- **Avoid Overtraining:** Increase weight and distance gradually to allow your body to adapt.
- **Listen to Your Body:** Pay attention to signs of fatigue and pain, and rest when needed.

Proper Warm-Up and Cool-Down

- **Dynamic Warm-Up:** Include movements like leg swings and arm circles to prepare your muscles.
- **Cool-Down:** Stretch major muscle groups after your ruck to aid recovery.

Foot Care

- **Prevent Blisters:** Use moisture-wicking socks and apply blister prevention products.
- **Footwear Fit:** Ensure your shoes or boots fit well and are broken in before long rucks.

Hydration and Nutrition

- **Stay Hydrated:** Drink water regularly, especially in hot weather.
- **Balanced Diet:** Maintain a diet rich in nutrients to support your training.

Weather Preparedness

- **Dress Appropriately:** Wear layers in cold weather and lightweight, breathable clothing in hot weather.
- **Sun Protection:** Use sunscreen, wear a hat, and sunglasses to protect against sun exposure.

Setting Realistic Goals

Setting realistic goals is crucial for sustained motivation and progress in rucking.

Goal Types

- **Short-Term Goals:** Focus on immediate objectives like completing a certain distance or improving your pace.
- **Long-Term Goals:** Aim for larger milestones such as participating in a rucking event or increasing your ruck weight significantly.

SMART Goals

- **Specific:** Clearly define what you want to achieve.
- **Measurable:** Ensure your goal can be quantified.
- **Achievable:** Set a goal that is realistic based on your current fitness level.
- **Relevant:** Choose goals that align with your overall fitness objectives.
- **Time-Bound:** Set a deadline for achieving your goal.

Tracking Progress

- **Regular Assessments:** Monitor your progress through regular check-ins and adjust your plan as needed.
- **Celebrate Milestones:** Acknowledge your achievements to stay motivated. # Training for Rucking Events

Preparing for rucking events requires a structured approach to training, nutrition, and mental preparation.

Training Plan

- **Build Endurance:** Gradually increase the distance and weight of your rucks.
- **Strength Training:** Incorporate exercises that enhance leg and core strength.
- **Cardiovascular Fitness:** Engage in cross-training activities like running and cycling.

Simulating Event Conditions

- **Terrain Training:** Train on similar terrain to what you will encounter during the event.
- **Weight Simulation:** Train with the same weight and gear you'll use during the event.

Nutrition and Hydration

- **Pre-Event Nutrition:** Focus on carbohydrate loading and balanced meals.
- **During Event:** Stay hydrated and consume energyboosting snacks.
- **Post-Event Recovery:** Rehydrate and eat a meal rich in protein and carbohydrates.

Mental Preparation

- **Set Goals:** Define performance and process goals for the event.
- **Visualization:** Use mental imagery to prepare for the event.
- **Positive Self-Talk:** Maintain a positive mindset and use affirmations.

Stories from the Field

Hearing real-life experiences from ruckers can provide inspiration and valuable insights.

Overcoming Challenges

- **Sarah's Journey:** A beginner who gradually built up her endurance and completed a 50K rucking event, demonstrating the importance of gradual training and mental resilience.

Teamwork and Camaraderie

- **Mike's Experience:** A veteran rucker who found that teamwork and support from fellow participants were crucial in completing a GORUCK Tough event.

Charity and Purpose

- **Laura's Motivation:** Participated in a Hike for Heroes event, driven by the cause she was supporting. Her story highlights the motivational power of participating in charity events.

Popular Rucking Challenges

Exploring popular rucking challenges can help you choose events that match your interests and abilities.

GORUCK Challenges

- **GORUCK Light, Tough, and Heavy:** Varying levels of difficulty, emphasizing teamwork, leadership, and endurance.

Hike for Heroes

- **Charitable Hikes:** Long-distance hikes to raise funds for military and first responder charities, adding a fundraising component to the physical challenge.

GoRuck Star Course

- **50-Miler:** A demanding event that involves navigating and covering 50 miles in 20 hours, requiring a combination of endurance and speed.

Ultimate Ruck Challenge

- **24-Hour Ruck:** Participants ruck as many miles as possible within 24 hours, testing mental toughness and endurance.

Final Thoughts

Rucking is a versatile and rewarding physical activity that offers numerous benefits for both physical and mental health. Whether you're a beginner taking your first steps or an experienced rucker preparing for a challenging event, the key is to approach rucking with a structured plan, the right gear, and a focus on safety and gradual progression. The stories and experiences of fellow ruckers highlight the sense of community and personal achievement that comes with this unique form of exercise. Embrace the journey, set realistic goals, and enjoy the numerous rewards that rucking has to offer. Happy rucking!